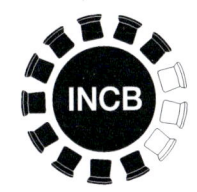

INTERNATIONAL NARCOTICS CONTROL BOARD

Report of the International Narcotics Control Board on the Availability of Internationally Controlled Drugs: Ensuring Adequate Access for Medical and Scientific Purposes

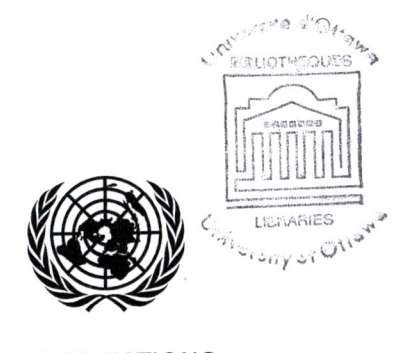

UNITED NATIONS
New York, 2011

E/INCB/2010/1/Supp.1

UNITED NATIONS PUBLICATION
Sales No. E.11.XI.7
ISBN: 978-92-1-148260-7

© United Nations: International Narcotics Control Board, January 2011. All rights reserved.

The designations employed and the presentation of material in this publication do not imply the expression of any opinion whatsoever on the part of the Secretariat of the United Nations concerning the legal status of any country, territory, city or area, or of its authorities, or concerning the delimitation of its frontiers or boundaries.

Countries and areas are referred to by the names that were in official use at the time the relevant data were collected.

Publishing production: English, Publishing and Library Section, United Nations Office at Vienna.

Preface

The objective of the international drug control conventions is to ensure adequate availability of narcotic drugs and psychotropic substances for medical and scientific purposes while ensuring that such drugs are not diverted for illicit purposes. The International Narcotics Control Board is mandated to monitor the implementation of this treaty objective, and has repeatedly voiced its concern about the disparate and inadequate access to controlled substances for medical and scientific purposes worldwide.

For many years, global consumption of narcotic drugs and psychotropic substances has been below the levels required for the most basic treatments. As a result of growing recognition of the therapeutic value of controlled substances, as well as the efforts of the international community, substantial increases in consumption have been achieved. However, while consumption levels have risen in several regions of the world, the bulk of the increase has occurred in a limited number of countries, particularly in three regions: Europe, North America and Oceania. Within some countries or regions, consumption levels have stagnated or even decreased. As long as these drugs remain inaccessible to the large majority of people around the world, patients will not be able to derive the health benefits to which they are entitled under the Universal Declaration of Human Rights.

For these reasons, the Board has decided to highlight this critical issue in a stand-alone supplement to its report for 2010. The supplement presents a thorough analysis of the global situation and regional variations in the consumption of internationally controlled substances, identifies the main impediments to adequate availability and provides recommendations on how the problem can be addressed.

Most narcotic drugs and psychotropic substances controlled under the international drug control treaties are indispensable in medical practice. Opioid analgesics, such as codeine and morphine, as well as semi-synthetic and synthetic opioids, are essential medicines for the treatment of pain. Psychotropic substances such as benzodiazepine-type anxiolytics and sedative-hypnotics and barbiturates are indispensable medications for the treatment of neurological and mental disorders. Pharmaceutical preparations containing internationally controlled substances play an essential role in medical treatment to relieve pain and suffering.

The international drug control treaties continue to be highly effective in preventing the diversion of drugs from licit to illicit markets and in protecting society from the consequences of dependence. However, in many countries equal attention has not been given to the other objective of the treaties — ensuring the adequate availability of controlled substances. Measures taken by Governments to prevent the abuse of and trafficking in narcotics drugs and psychotropic substances must not hinder the utilization of such drugs for medical treatment. Governments need to meet the dual objective of the international drug control treaties, namely, preventing the diversion and abuse of internationally controlled substances while ensuring their availability for legitimate use. This balance should be reflected in national drug control laws and regulations.

The first step towards improving access to these essential drugs for medical and scientific purposes is to identify the impediments, which are manifold. While economic considerations may play a role with regard to high-cost medications, low cost preparations do exist, and examples of countries making use of such preparations demonstrate that economic impediments can be overcome. Systemic and regulatory problems may lead to inadequate availability of controlled substances.

To assist Governments in eliminating these impediments, the present supplement includes a wide range of practical recommendations that can be tailored to each national situation. I truly hope that Governments will make full use of this report to assess the situation in their countries and to implement the relevant recommendations. Unless remedial measures are urgently implemented, the gap between high-consumption and low-consumption countries may widen, with unnecessary pain and suffering continuing in many countries.

Hamid **Ghodse**
President
International Narcotics Control Board

Summary

The International Narcotics Control Board was invited by the Commission on Narcotic Drugs at its fifty-third session, in March 2010, to include in its report for 2010 information on the availability of internationally controlled substances for medical requirements. The Board is aware of the growing interest of the World Health Organization, other intergovernmental bodies and non-governmental organizations in this matter. In recognition of its importance, the Board has decided to devote a supplement to its annual report to this subject. This format allows the Board to provide adequate information on the present situation, globally and regionally, to highlight major impediments and to formulate recommendations to improve the availability of internationally controlled substances for medical and scientific purposes. A detailed analysis is contained in the Board's technical publications on narcotic drugs and psychotropic substances.

CONTENTS

		Page
	Preface	iii
Chapter I.	Introduction	1
Chapter II.	Action taken by the Board to ensure adequate availability	5
Chapter III.	Supply of opiate raw materials and opioids	9
	A. Supply of opiate raw materials	10
	B. Supply of opioids controlled under the 1961 Convention	11
	C. Supply of opioids currently controlled under the 1971 Convention	12
	D. Supply of stimulants controlled under the 1971 Convention	13
	E. Supply of benzodiazepines and barbiturates controlled under the 1971 Convention	13
Chapter IV.	Availability of medicines containing internationally controlled substances	15
	A. Availability of opioid analgesics controlled under the 1961 Convention	18
	B. Opioids controlled under the 1971 Convention	26
	C. Anti-epileptics	28
	D. Stimulants in Schedule II of the 1971 Convention that are used for the treatment of attention deficit disorder	29
	E. Stimulants in Schedule IV of the 1971 Convention that are used as anorectics	30
	F. Benzodiazepines	32
Chapter V.	Achieving a balance between ensuring availability of internationally controlled substances for medical and scientific purposes and preventing their diversion and abuse	43
	A. Impediments to availability of opioid analgesics	44
	B. Availability of internationally controlled substances above levels required for sound medical practice	47
	C. Ensuring adequate availability in emergency situations	49
Chapter VI.	Conclusions and recommendations	51
Annexes		
	I. Tables on consumption of opioid analgesics in regions	59
	II. Joint letter from the President of the International Narcotics Control Board and the Chair of the United Nations Development Group	69
	III. Follow-up joint letter from the President of the International Narcotics Control Board and the Chair of the United Nations Development Group	71
	IV. Letter from the President of the International Narcotics Control Board to all countries	73

Introduction

1. Ensuring the availability of internationally controlled substances for treatment in accordance with article 9 of the Single Convention on Narcotics Drugs of 1961 (1961 Convention),[1] as amended by the 1972 Protocol,[2] and the preamble of the 1971 Convention on Psychotropic Substances (1971 Convention)[3] is a mandate of the International Narcotics Control Board.

2. By becoming parties to the international drug control conventions, Governments have accepted the obligation to introduce the provisions of those treaties into their national legislation and to implement them. The International Narcotics Control Board is the body established by the 1961 Convention that is responsible for monitoring the compliance of Governments with the international drug control treaties and for providing support to Governments in this respect.

3. The conventions established a control regime to serve a dual purpose: to ensure the availability of controlled substances for medical and scientific ends while preventing the illicit production of, trafficking in and abuse of such substances. The 1961 Convention, while recognizing that addiction to narcotic drugs constitutes a serious evil for the individual and is fraught with social and economic danger to humankind, affirms that the medical use of narcotic drugs continues to be indispensable for the relief of pain and suffering and that adequate provision must be made to ensure the availability of narcotic drugs for such purposes. Equally, the 1971 Convention recognizes that, while the parties to the Convention were determined to prevent and combat abuse of and trafficking in psychotropic substances, their use for medical and scientific purposes is indispensable and that their availability for such purposes should not be unduly restricted. The implementation of the international drug control treaties by parties is monitored by the Board, whose responsibilities under article 9 of the 1961 Convention expressly include the responsibility to ensure the availability of narcotic drugs for medical and scientific purposes.

4. The international drug control treaties recognize that narcotic drugs and psychotropic substances are indispensable for medical and scientific purposes. However, despite numerous efforts by the Board and the World Health Organization (WHO), as well as non-governmental organizations, their availability in much of the world remains very limited, depriving many patients of essential medicines. The Board continues to monitor the worldwide availability of narcotic drugs and psychotropic substances and has made their availability one of the main topics of its dialogue with Governments on adequate treaty implementation.

---

[1] United Nations, *Treaty Series*, vol. 520, No. 7515.
[2] Ibid., vol. 976, No. 14152.
[3] Ibid., vol. 1019, No. 14956.

REPORT ON THE AVAILABILITY OF INTERNATIONALLY CONTROLLED DRUGS

5. Narcotic drugs such as morphine, fentanyl and oxycodone are opioid analgesics effective for the treatment of moderate and severe pain. Data from 2009 show that more than 90 per cent of the global consumption of these opioid analgesics occurred in Australia, Canada, New Zealand, the United States of America and several European countries. This means that their availability was very limited in many countries and in entire regions. Although medical science has the capacity to provide relief for most forms of moderate to severe pain, over 80 per cent of the world population will have insufficient analgesia, or no analgesia at all, if they suffer from such pain.[4]

Figure 1. Distribution of morphine consumption, 2009

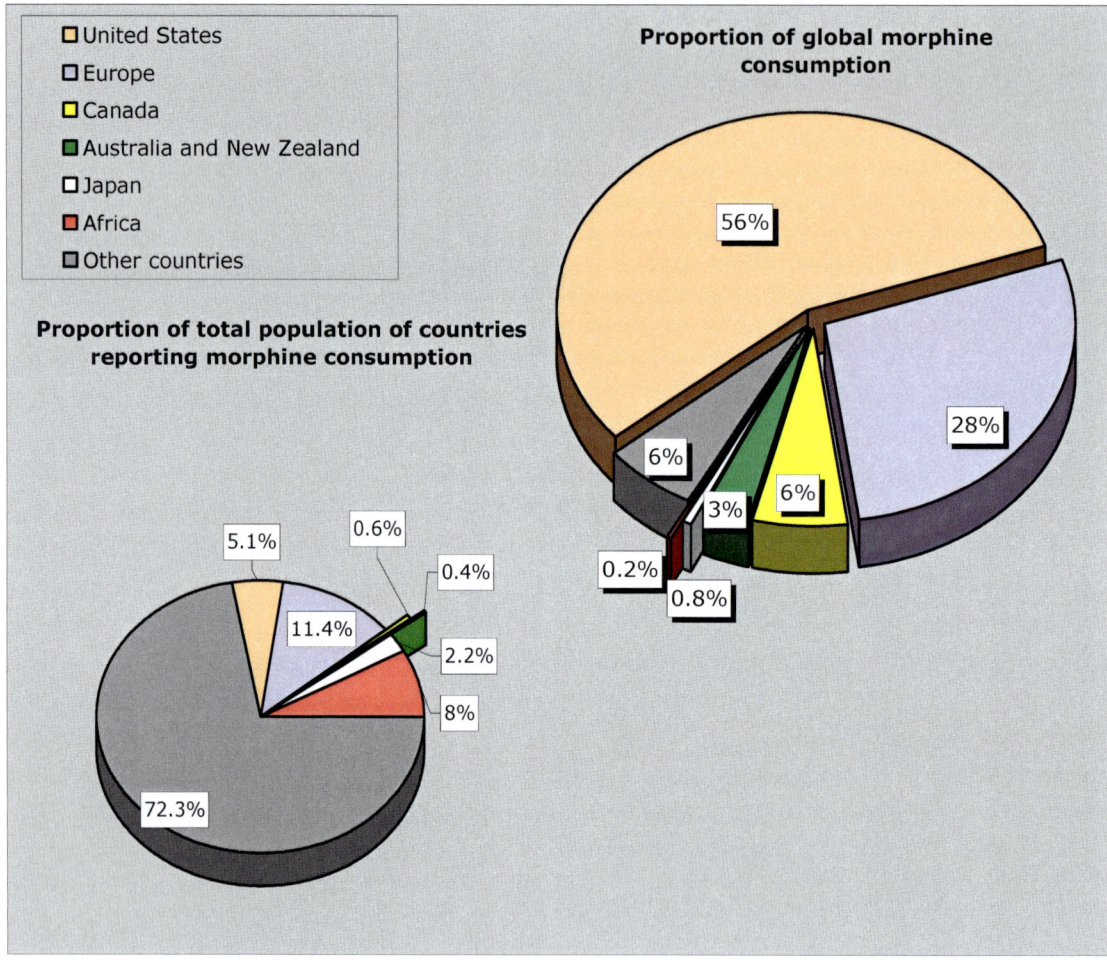

6. Similar disparities exist for the consumption levels of psychotropic substances, although their identification is more difficult, as the 1971 Convention does not require Governments to provide consumption data on such substances to the Board.

7. Taking into account that the global supply of opiate raw materials is sufficient for the production of opioid analgesics such as morphine, codeine and other alkaloids, and does not

---

[4] There are a number of safe and effective methods to treat pain. Opioid analgesics continue to be the mainstay for the relief of moderate to severe pain.

constitute a barrier to the availability of narcotic drugs, it should be possible to significantly improve this situation through appropriate action by Governments. However, many other barriers to adequate availability, identified and highlighted by the Board in the past, continue to exist. The present supplement to the report of the Board for 2010 focuses on efforts undertaken to ensure adequate availability, developments over recent years and the current levels of availability of narcotic drugs and psychotropic substances, and provides recommendations for action to be taken at the international and national levels.

Action taken by the Board to ensure adequate availability

8. The Board, acting under the mandate assigned to it by the Conventions, was among the first to issue a warning that availability of narcotic drugs was not ensured in a majority of countries. More than 20 years ago the Board became aware of this problem, being in a singular position to assess consumption in various countries. The 1961 Convention requires Governments to submit to the Board annual statistical data, including data on the consumption of narcotic drugs. Consumption data submitted by Governments are analysed by the Board and then published in its annual technical publication on narcotic drugs. While reporting on consumption of psychotropic substances is not required by the 1971 Convention, consumption is calculated on the basis of other statistical data provided to the Board[5] and is published in the annual technical publication on psychotropic substances.

9. The regular analysis of consumption data, particularly regarding narcotic drugs, convinced the Board that the level of consumption of narcotic drugs was very low in a number of countries. Therefore, in 1989, the Board, in cooperation with WHO, assessed the medical need for opiates in the world. They found that medical needs for opiates were not being fully satisfied, in particular for the treatment of cancer pain.

10. The Board found that only a few countries had established effective systems for assessing medical needs. A number of interrelated factors were identified as important impediments. Laws and regulations, and their administration or interpretation, unduly impeded the availability of opiates. Lack of resources in the health-care system prevented the optimal availability and use of opiates. Fear of addiction among professionals and the public was also a deterrent to the appropriate medical prescription of opiates. In addition, lack of up-to-date professional training impeded the adequate use of opioids to treat pain.

11. The findings of this study were published in the Board's special report for 1989 on the demand for and supply of opiates for medical and scientific needs.[6] The Board made a number of recommendations to Governments to help them to minimize or overcome many of the impediments to making opiates available for medical needs. Governments were requested to examine their methods of assessing medical needs for opiates; evaluate their health-care systems and laws and regulations for impediments to opiate availability; develop plans of action to facilitate the availability of opiates for all appropriate conditions; and establish national policies, guidelines and professional education on the rational medical use of opiates.

---

[5] Data on manufacture, imports, exports and stocks of psychotropic substances.
[6] United Nations publication, Sales No. E.89.XI.5.

12. Five years later, in 1994, the Board examined the effectiveness of the international drug control treaties in a supplement to its annual report, entitled *Effectiveness of the International Drug Control Treaties*.[7] In its evaluation the Board concluded that the treaty objective of ensuring an adequate supply of narcotic drugs, especially opiates used for medical purposes, had not been universally achieved.

13. Therefore, in 1995, the Board published another special report, entitled *Availability of Opiates for Medical Needs*,[8] which included specific recommendations to Governments, the United Nations International Drug Control Programme, the Commission on Narcotic Drugs, WHO, international and regional drug control, health and humanitarian organizations and educational institutions and non-governmental health-care organizations, including the International Association for the Study of Pain, and other health-care representatives. The recommendations of the special report are still valid. Furthermore, chapter I of the report of the Board for 1999[9] was dedicated to the issue of availability of narcotic analgesics. The Board identified in that chapter, inter alia, constraints and impediments to the adequate availability of opioids for the treatment of pain and made recommendations to Governments for corrective action. As internationally controlled drugs were overused in some countries, leading to prescription drug abuse and related problems, chapter I of the report of the Board for 2000[10] dealt with overconsumption of internationally controlled drugs and recommended a balanced approach in their use.

14. One tool to assess whether countries improve availability levels, or at least are aware of the problem and show the intention to improve, is the analysis of the estimates for narcotic drugs, which all countries submit to the Board. The Board regularly contacts countries with missing or particularly low estimates in order to ensure adequate availability of opioids for the treatment of pain. This practice was formalized in November 1999, when the Board started selecting certain groups of countries with low levels of consumption of opioid analgesics (mainly morphine) and with common characteristics.[11] In 2004 the Board contacted four countries[12] that had significantly increased their consumption levels and requested information on the policies and activities they considered the main causes for their growing consumption of opioid analgesics, in particular morphine, in order to make this information available to countries that needed to improve their consumption levels.

15. The matter was repeatedly brought to the attention of Governments in circular letters to all countries and specific letters to individual countries. In August 2001, a joint letter from the President of the Board and the Chair of the United Nations Development Group was sent to all resident coordinators of the United Nations system at the country level, urging them, inter alia, to be aware of underconsumption and the lack of medicaments available for the treatment of severe pain in many developing countries (see annex II). This request was confirmed in February 2005, in a follow-up joint letter from the President of the Board and the Chair of the United Nations Development Group (see annex III). In April 2006, the President of the Board emphasized in a letter to all

---

[7] United Nations publication, Sales No. E.95.XI.5.
[8] United Nations publication, Sales No. E.96.XI.6.
[9] United Nations publication, Sales No. E.00.XI.1. United Nations publication, Sales No. E.96.XI.6.
[10] United Nations publication, Sales No. E.01.XI.1.
[11] Main characteristics for selection: no estimates for morphine; large population and very low level of consumption of morphine; very high cancer rate and low level of consumption of analgesics; functioning control administration but low level of availability; high-income countries outside Europe and North America with inadequate availability.
[12] Brazil, Canada, France, United States of America.

countries the difficulties of access to narcotic drugs and psychotropic substances for needy patients and encouraged Governments to take measures to ensure the inclusion of the subject of rational use of drugs in the curricula of the appropriate university faculties (see annex IV).[13]

16. The subject of availability of opioids for the treatment of pain is discussed with individual Governments during all missions of the Board. The letters of recommendation sent to Governments after the missions include, if appropriate, specific recommendations on the availability of opioids for the treatment of pain. Equally, the WHO guidelines on achieving balance in national opioids control policy[14] are always included in the information material provided to competent authorities during Board missions.

17. The Board regularly includes the subject of the availability of narcotic drugs in speeches at meetings of intergovernmental bodies, such as the twentieth special session of the General Assembly, sessions of the Commission on Narcotic Drugs, the Economic and Social Council and World Health Assembly, and regional meetings of international organizations. In March 2010, at the fifty-third session of the Commission on Narcotic Drugs, the discussion of availability resulted in Commission resolution 53/4, entitled "Promoting adequate availability of internationally controlled licit drugs for medical and scientific purposes while preventing their diversion and abuse".

18. WHO is the main partner of the Board in activities to increase the availability of opioids for the treatment of pain. Specific cooperative activities between the Board and WHO include the promotion by the Board of the WHO guidelines on achieving balance in national opioids control policy; the establishment of a working group on availability in 2003, which prepared a proposal for strengthening working relationships between the Board and WHO with regard to the availability of narcotic medicines and promoting rational use of psychotropic medicines; and cooperating in the WHO global strategy against pain, aimed at providing assistance to countries in, inter alia, building capacity and raising awareness in the area of using opioids in pain treatment.

19. The World Health Assembly, in its resolution WHA58.22, and the Economic and Social Council, in its resolution 2005/25, invited WHO and the Board to examine the feasibility of an assistance mechanism to facilitate the adequate treatment of pain using opioid analgesics. WHO and the Board reviewed documents and studies on the availability of opioid analgesics at the country level and examined activities conducted and planned by various bodies to assist Governments to ensure the availability of those medicines for legitimate medical use. They concluded that although there was no shortage of licitly produced opioid analgesic raw material worldwide and global licit consumption of opioids had increased substantially in the past two decades, access to opioid analgesics continued to be difficult in many countries, owing to several constraints.

20. WHO and the Board found that an assistance mechanism to facilitate adequate treatment of pain using opioid analgesics was feasible. Therefore, WHO started the preparation of the Access to Controlled Medications Programme and developed the framework of that Programme in consultation with the Board. The Programme is implemented by WHO. The Board actively promotes

---

[13] Those three letters are also posted on the Board's website at www.incb.org/incb/en/other-issues_correspondence.html.
[14] World Health Organization, document WHO/EDM/QSM/2000.4.

the Programme during its missions, in speeches on the subject of availability and through specific references and recommendations in its annual reports.

21.   However, while consumption of narcotic drugs for medical purposes had increased significantly in some countries, owing inter alia, to the efforts of the Board, the level of availability of substances controlled under international conventions remained low and inadequate in most countries. The Board therefore concluded that the promotion of a better understanding of the provisions of the international drug control treaties was required. One major part of this effort is the provision of assistance to Governments in establishing more realistic estimates of requirements for medications containing controlled substances. The Board and WHO are at present jointly developing guidelines on estimating requirements for substances under international control. This initiative is intended to identify methods to be applied by countries to arrive at adequate estimates for narcotic drugs, assessments for psychotropic substances and estimates for some precursors for medical purposes.

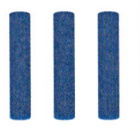

III. Supply of opiate raw materials and opioids

22. "Opiate" is the term generally used to designate drugs derived from opium and their chemically related derivatives, such as the semi-synthetic alkaloids, while "opioid" is a more general term for both natural and synthetic drugs with morphine-like properties, although the chemical structure may differ from that of morphine.

23. The natural alkaloids contained in opium or poppy straw that are under international control are morphine, codeine, thebaine and oripavine. Morphine and codeine are under international control because of their potential for abuse, while thebaine and oripavine are under such control because of their convertibility into opioids subject to abuse. Morphine is the prototype of natural opiates and many opioids, and, because of its strong analgesic potency, it is used as a reference parameter for comparative purposes.

24. Opioids are used mostly for their analgesic properties to treat severe pain (fentanyl, hydromorphone, methadone, morphine and pethidine), moderate to severe pain (buprenorphine[15] and oxycodone) and mild to moderate pain (codeine, dihydrocodeine and dextropropoxyphene). They are also used to induce or supplement anaesthesia (fentanyl and fentanyl analogues such as alfentanil and remifentanil), as cough suppressants (codeine, dihydrocodeine and, to a lesser extent, pholcodine and ethylmorphine) and to treat addiction to opioids (buprenorphine and methadone).

Main opioids controlled under the 1961 Convention and buprenorphine[a]

Natural alkaloids	Semi-synthetic opioids	Synthetic opioids
Morphine	Dihydrocodeine	Dextropropoxyphene
Codeine	Ethylmorphine	Diphenoxylate
Thebaine	Heroin	Fentanyl and analogues
Oripavine	Hydrocodone	Ketobemidone
	Hydromorphone	Methadone
	Oxycodone	Pethidine
	Pholcodine	Tilidine
	Buprenorphine	

[a] Buprenorphine is controlled under the 1971 Convention.

25. Semi-synthetic opioids are made by relatively simple chemical modifications of natural opiates, such as morphine, codeine and thebaine. Some examples of those derivatives are dihydrocodeine, ethylmorphine, heroin, oxycodone and pholcodine. Synthetic opioids are fully

---
[15] Buprenorphine is controlled under the 1971 Convention.

man-made and not related to opiates, although they have similar effects when used in treatment. The most commonly used synthetic opioids include fentanyl and fentanyl analogues, methadone and pethidine.

A. Supply of opiate raw materials

26. Opiates consumed by patients for medical treatment are obtained from opiate raw materials (opium, poppy straw and concentrate of poppy straw). Adequate availability of opiate raw materials for the manufacture of opiates is therefore a precondition for ensuring the adequate availability of opiates used for medical and scientific purposes.

27. Pursuant to the 1961 Convention and the relevant resolutions of the Commission on Narcotic Drugs and the Economic and Social Council, the Board examines on a regular basis developments affecting the supply of and demand for opiate raw materials. The Board endeavours, in cooperation with Governments, to maintain a lasting balance between supply and demand. When analysing the situation regarding the supply of and demand for opiate raw materials, the Board uses information from Governments of countries producing opiate raw materials, as well as from Governments of countries where those materials are utilized for the manufacture of opiates or substances not controlled under the 1961 Convention. A detailed analysis of the present situation with regard to the supply of opiate raw materials and demand for those materials worldwide is contained in the 2010 report of the Board on narcotic drugs.[16]

28. Global stocks of opiate raw materials should cover global demand for about one year to ensure the availability of opiates used for medical and scientific purposes in the event of an unexpected decline in production resulting from, for example, adverse weather conditions in producing countries.[17] At the end of 2009, global stocks of opiate raw materials rich in morphine were sufficient to cover global demand for 12 months. Global stocks of opiate raw materials rich in thebaine were sufficient to cover global demand for slightly less than 12 months; however, that was compensated for by the high level of stocks of thebaine and opiates derived from thebaine, which were sufficient at the end of 2009 to cover global demand for those opiates for about 14 months.

29. According to information available to the Board, in 2010 global production of opiate raw materials rich in morphine was greater than the utilization of those materials. The global supply (stocks and production) of opiate raw materials rich in morphine was fully sufficient to cover global demand. For 2011, Governments of producing countries are planning to further extend the area cultivated with opium poppy rich in morphine.

30. As for opiate raw materials rich in thebaine, information available to the Board indicates that global production exceeded global demand in 2010. Total stocks of opiate raw materials rich in thebaine were sufficient to cover global demand for less than one year. The plans of the producing countries indicate that global production of opiate raw materials rich in thebaine will exceed global

---

[16] Narcotic Drugs: Estimated World Requirements for 2011 — Statistics for 2009 (United Nations publication, Sales No. T.11.XI.2).
[17] *Report of the International Narcotics Control Board for 2005* (United Nations publication, Sales No. E.06.XI.2), para. 85.

demand in 2011 as well. Total stocks of opiate raw materials rich in thebaine are therefore expected to increase to a level that can cover about 14 months of demand. The global supply (stocks and production) of opiate raw materials rich in thebaine will continue to be sufficient to fully cover global demand.

31. Global demand for opiate raw materials rich in morphine and rich in thebaine is expected to rise in the future as well. It is anticipated that, as a result of the activities of the Board and WHO to ensure the adequate availability of opioid analgesics, global demand for opiates and opiate raw materials will continue to rise.

B. Supply of opioids controlled under the 1961 Convention

32. As in the case of steadily rising production of opiate raw materials, manufacture of opioids has also progressively increased in the last 20 years. The manufacture of morphine and the major synthetic and semi-synthetic opioids has increased fivefold in the last 20 years, with the synthetic and semi-synthetic opioids recording higher growth rates than morphine. This development is strongly related to the increasing demand for certain narcotic drugs, as well as the development of new products.

Figure 2.   Growth in manufacture of opioids, 1989-2009

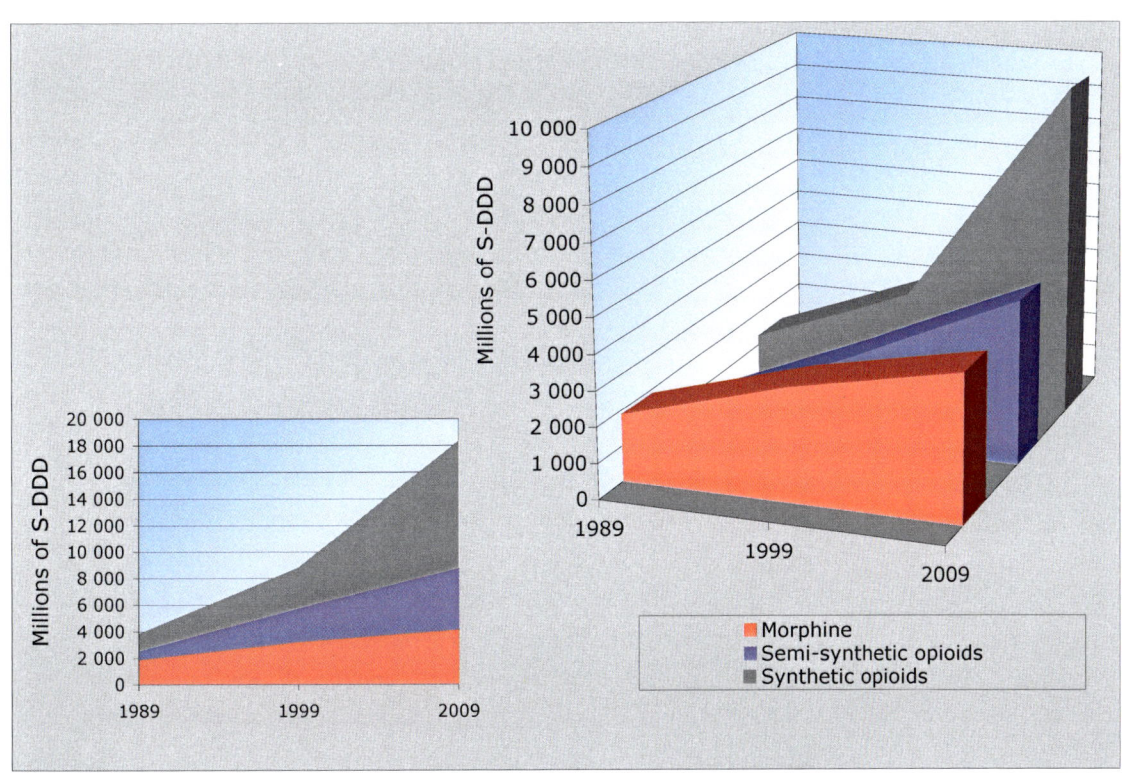

33. Figure 2 shows the aggregated growth in manufacture of morphine and synthetic and semi-synthetic opioids over a period of 20 years. The term S-DDD (defined daily doses for statistical purposes) represents a technical unit of measurement used for statistical analysis and is not a recommended prescription dose. This unit of measurement is used whenever narcotic drugs or psychotropic substances with different levels of potency, and therefore different levels of daily dosage in treatment, are aggregated to show the quantities available for a group of substances in a comparable unit of measurement.

34. Particularly strong growth rates were recorded for fentanyl, which has become the most manufactured synthetic opioid when amounts are expressed in S-DDD. When used as an analgesic, fentanyl is about 100 times as potent as morphine and is used for anaesthesia in very small doses (for example, 0.005-0.1 mg in injectable form). The use of controlled-release patches of fentanyl for the treatment of severe pain, containing higher dosages and used for up to three days, has been increasing in all parts of the world resulting in increased manufacture of fentanyl. Methadone is also manufactured in much larger quantities than it was 20 years ago, although mostly for use in substitution treatment. The manufacture of the semi-synthetic drugs hydrocodone, hydromorphone, oxycodone and oxymorphone has also shown very high rates of increase. International trade in narcotic drugs increased comparably: fivefold for morphine, by nearly 300 times for fentanyl and by more than 130 times for oxycodone.

35. Those are impressive growth rates for manufacture of and international trade in narcotic drugs. However, the major reason for those rates was the strong increase in imports in some high-consumption countries, while most other countries either increased imports to a much lesser extent or started out from such low levels that even very high increase rates did not translate into large absolute quantities. Moreover, out of 211 countries and territories, 17 did not import any morphine, 22 did not import any fentanyl and 9 did not import any opioids.

36. Data available to the Board show that the manufacture of morphine and the synthetic and semi-synthetic opioids at present is fully adequate to satisfy global demand. In addition, ongoing research into new applications and preparations allows the manufacture of new medications that are easier and more comfortable to use. At the same time, other, less costly types of preparations continue to be manufactured. Increasing demand for products in different price ranges can be covered by the pharmaceutical industry. The supply side for opioids can therefore not be considered an obstacle to the adequate availability of narcotic drugs.

C. Supply of opioids currently controlled under the 1971 Convention

37. Global manufacture of buprenorphine has also risen fivefold in the last 20 years and has reached a level comparable to that of the major opioids. It increased sharply in the late 1990s, as the substance started to be used in higher doses for the treatment of opioid addiction, and another sharp rise is evident since 2006. Equally, international trade in the substance increased sharply, and 80 countries reported imports of buprenorphine in the period from 2007 to 2009. However, the number of countries importing buprenorphine is much smaller than the number of countries

importing at least one of the main opioids. There is much less manufacture and trade of pentazocine, another major synthetic analgesic controlled under the 1971 Convention, which did not show a comparable trend. While there are fluctuations in manufacture and trade, no steady increase rate is discernible.

D. Supply of stimulants controlled under the 1971 Convention

38. Stimulants included in Schedule II are manufactured in about a dozen countries and imported by a further 90 countries. Particularly high growth rates in manufacture in the last 20 years were recorded for methylphenidate (16-fold) and dexamfetamine (2.5-fold), while manufacture of amfetamine[18] reached a peak in 1998 and has been declining since. International trade of stimulants in Schedule II also increased, more so for methylphenidate than for the amphetamines. During the last 10 years the manufacture and trade of stimulants in Schedule IV, mostly used as anorectics in anti-obesity treatment, remained at roughly the same level. The level of manufacture of the whole group, comprising 14 substances and expressed in S DDD, is below the level of manufacture of the major opioids.

E. Supply of benzodiazepines and barbiturates controlled under the 1971 Convention

39. The manufacture and trade of benzodiazepine-type anxiolytics and sedative hypnotics, after strong growth rates 20 years ago, have reached a plateau (between 20 billion and 30 billion S-DDD for anxiolytics; between 5 billion and 9 billion S-DDD for sedative-hypnotics) at which they fluctuate. Manufacture of barbiturates has also remained stable during the last 10 years. The significant regional differences in international trade in anxiolytics and sedative-hypnotics remained, and in certain regions that had always reported only very low levels of such imports, further reductions were noted (mostly African countries, but also in some parts of Asia). The two most traded psychotropic substances in terms of the number of countries importing are diazepam, a benzodiazepine-type anxiolytic, and phenobarbital, a barbiturate, both of them imported by more than 160 countries. The most manufactured psychotropic substance when expressed in S-DDD is the benzodiazepine-type anxiolytic alprazolam.

---

[18] Most of the substances in the schedules of the 1971 Convention are listed by their international non-proprietary names (INN). The INN system was developed by WHO to facilitate the identification of pharmaceutical substances or active pharmaceutical ingredients. (Those names are used in the technical report of the Board on psychotropic substances.) If no INN exists, the substances are listed in the schedules under "other non-proprietary or trivial names".
To most native speakers of English, the INN of many of the substances in Schedule II of the 1971 Convention appear to be misspellings: amfetamine, dexamfetamine, levamfetamine, metamfetamine, metamfetamine racemate. In the present report, the "other non-proprietary or trivial names" of those substances, which are more common, are used: amphetamine, dexamphetamine, levamphetamine, methamphetamine, methamphetamine racemate.

IV. Availability of medicines containing internationally controlled substances

40. Adequate supply of licitly produced opiate raw materials and of the end products manufactured using those raw materials, as well as increasing manufacture of psychotropic substances, does not necessarily lead to adequate supply of medicines containing those substances for the end-user, the patient. Access to opioid-based medicines, as well as other medicines containing substances under international control, is limited or almost non-existent in many countries. That discrepancy has been discussed repeatedly not only by the Board but also by the Commission on Narcotic Drugs.

41. As mentioned above, the Commission on Narcotic Drugs, in its resolution 53/4, entitled "Promoting adequate availability of internationally controlled licit drugs for medical and scientific purposes while preventing their diversion and abuse", recalled the 1961 Convention as amended by the 1972 Protocol, as well as the 1971 Convention. That resolution reflects the recognition in both Conventions that internationally controlled substances are indispensable for medical treatment and scientific purposes. In that resolution the Commission recalled that the availability of internationally controlled substances should not be unduly restricted and that provision must be made to ensure their availability for medical and scientific purposes.

42. In the same resolution, the Commission invited the Board to include in its annual report for 2010 information on the consumption of narcotic drugs and psychotropic substances used for medical and scientific purposes worldwide, including an analysis of impediments to their adequate availability, actions to be taken to overcome those impediments and, when available, specific information about the status of and progress made by countries. Pursuant to that resolution, the Board carried out an analysis of global developments and regional patterns of consumption of opioid analgesics based on statistics furnished by Governments. It also analysed the global developments and regional patterns of consumption of psychotropic substances.[19]

43. In order to show discrepancies between regions, as well as between countries within regions, the Board's technical publication on narcotic drugs provides regional tables on consumption levels of opioid analgesics, in addition to the global table on average consumption of narcotic drugs (table XIV of the technical publication on narcotic drugs). Governments are required to provide to the Board, in their annual statistics on narcotic drugs, data on the consumption of opioid analgesics. Countries have been collecting such data for many years, but not all of them have developed adequate methods of assessing their requirements. The Board has created the concept of "defined daily doses for statistical purposes (S-DDD) consumed per million inhabitants per day",

---

[19] Calculated on the basis of statistical data furnished to the Board on manufacture, imports, exports and stocks.

which it uses when compiling and comparing statistics on the consumption of substances with different potency levels, such as opioid analgesics.

44. In the absence of a universally agreed expert opinion on adequate levels of consumption, the Board has internally, for administrative purposes, set some minimum standards to use when examining estimates of annual requirements for narcotic drugs submitted by countries. The Board has identified levels of consumption that it considers to be inadequate (consumption of opioid analgesics in quantities between 100 and 200 S-DDD per million inhabitants per day) or very inadequate (consumption of opioid analgesics in quantities equal to or less than 100 S-DDD). If those levels were to be used as a benchmark, 21 countries would have inadequate consumption levels and more than 100 other countries would have very inadequate consumption levels, most of them in Africa. In May 2004, the Board adopted an amendment to the rules for establishing estimates, which allowed for the raising of the estimates of certain essential narcotic drugs by the Board in case the existing estimates were considered inappropriately low.

45. In its resolution 53/4 the Commission on Narcotic Drugs invited the Board to present to the Commission information on the consumption of psychotropic substances used for medical and scientific purposes worldwide, to promote their adequate availability. However, Governments are not obliged to submit data on the consumption of psychotropic substances. The Board has found it useful in the past to calculate approximate consumption levels for psychotropic substances based on the statistical information on those substances that Governments have submitted to the Board in their annual statistics on psychotropic substances, to show global trends and, when data appear to be consistent and reliable, to identify unusual consumption patterns. As stated in the technical report of the Board on psychotropic substances, caution should be exercised when drawing conclusions on the actual level of consumption of psychotropic substances, at the global level as well as in specific countries, as data reported by Governments on the manufacture of and trade in psychotropic substances may not be complete or may not cover all substances. Calculated consumption levels tend to be particularly inaccurate for manufacturing countries. The calculated consumption levels are published in table IV of the technical report on psychotropic substances.

46. In the past, the analysis of calculated consumption levels of psychotropic substances often focused on consistently high levels of consumption that might not be medically justified and might lead to the diversion and abuse of the substances in question. However, the Board was aware that the very low levels of consumption of psychotropic substances observed in some countries might reflect the fact that those substances were almost inaccessible to certain segments of the population and that those substances, or counterfeit medicaments allegedly containing those substances, might therefore appear on unregulated markets to cover the unmet needs. It should also be taken into consideration that consumption levels for psychotropic substances vary greatly between countries and regions, because of differences in medical practice and related variations in prescription patterns. Comparisons between countries and regions can be made only with great care, especially since, for certain psychotropic substances, other psychotropic substances or non-psychotropic substances may be used as substitutes, which should be taken into account when reviewing the availability of those psychotropic substances.

47. The Board notes that on numerous occasions Governments have strengthened the international control regime for psychotropic substances by agreeing to provide additional data to

the Board, such as assessments of annual requirements for those substances and details on trade in substances in Schedules III and IV of the 1971 Convention and on stocks held by manufacturers. Since such data were not considered essential when the 1971 Convention was adopted, it was the Economic and Social Council that, in various resolutions,[20] introduced the requirement to collect and submit to the Board the above-mentioned additional information on psychotropic substances. Although this additional reporting is not yet universal, the Board appreciates the fact that most Governments submit the additional information pursuant to the resolutions of the Economic and Social Council and offers training for the national authorities responsible for completing and returning the forms.

48. In the opinion of the Board, it is again time for Governments to agree to voluntarily provide it with information not foreseen under the 1971 Convention but essential for the implementation of Commission on Narcotic Drugs resolution 53/4 so that the Board will be in a position to analyse trends in the consumption of psychotropic substances. Reliable data on the consumption of psychotropic substances will also be needed to assess the effectiveness of any measures taken in accordance with Commission resolution 53/4. The Board therefore strongly recommends that Governments consider providing it with data on the consumption of psychotropic substances, to enable the Board to comply with Commission resolution 53/4 and, ultimately, to promote the adequate availability of psychotropic substances used for medical and scientific purposes while preventing the diversion and abuse of those substances.

49. For the reasons mentioned above, the quality of data on the consumption of psychotropic substances is not comparable with the quality of data on the consumption of narcotic drugs. It is therefore more difficult to provide a meaningful analysis of the consumption levels for psychotropic substances. Moreover, in most countries psychotropic substances are used much more in medical treatment than narcotic drugs. To analyse the consumption patterns of psychotropic substances, the Board therefore uses the concept of S-DDD consumed per thousand inhabitants per day to compare and compile statistics of substances of different potency. Therefore, the information below is divided into information on consumption levels of opioid analgesics and information on analgesics controlled under the 1971 Convention, as well as information on other groups of psychotropic substances.

50. The situation with regard to the adequacy of consumption levels for psychotropic substances is similar to the situation with regard to the adequacy of consumption levels for narcotic drugs: there is no agreement among experts regarding the level of per capita consumption of any of the groups of psychotropic substances that is implied by "adequate availability".

51. The Commission on Narcotic Drugs, in its resolution 53/4, affirmed that the international drug control conventions sought to achieve a balance between ensuring the availability of narcotic drugs and psychotropic substances under international control for medical and scientific purposes and preventing their diversion and abuse. In the same resolution the Commission acknowledged that an increase in the licit supply of internationally controlled substances might increase the risk of diversion and abuse of those substances. The present supplement includes information on the consumption levels for certain groups of substances that may be considered too high. It is apparent

---

[20] Resolutions 1981/7, 1985/15, 1987/30 and 1991/44.

that in a few countries with high levels of consumption, narcotic analgesics are the main drug abuse problem and that the abuse of prescription drugs is increasing.

A. Availability of opioid analgesics controlled under the 1961 Convention

52. In the period 1989-2009, global consumption of opioid analgesics used for the treatment of moderate and severe pain increased considerably. For example, global consumption of morphine increased sevenfold. The increase was more dramatic for certain opioids under international control, such as fentanyl (100-fold) and oxycodone (26-fold). The increase was significantly higher in some regions than in others.[21] Within each region, the increase in consumption was greater in some countries than in others, and there continued to be large differences in the consumption levels of different countries. Consumption levels in regions, countries and territories are reflected in the tables in annex I.

Figure 3. All regions: average consumption of opioid analgesics, 1987-1989, 1997-1999 and 2007-2009

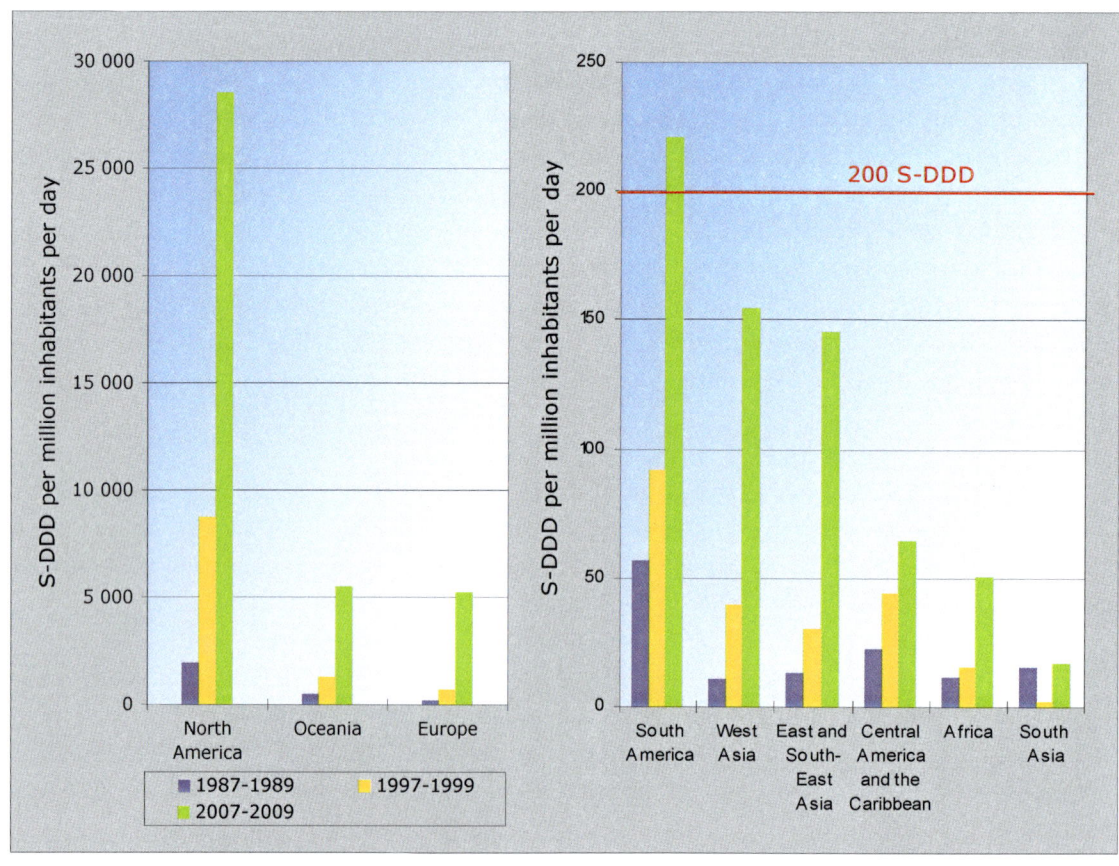

---

[21] Figures 3-13 provide information on the development in consumption levels of opioid analgesics globally and regionally over the last 20 years. Due to the significant differences in consumption levels, the scales used in the graphs are different.

AVAILABILITY OF MEDICINES CONTAINING INTERNATIONALLY CONTROLLED SUBSTANCES

53. The highest levels of consumption for opioid analgesics have been recorded in North American and European countries and Australia and New Zealand. In a large proportion of countries in Europe and North America the levels of consumption for opioid analgesics rose substantially in the period 2000-2009. Canada and the United States had the highest levels of consumption for opioid analgesics in the world. Those two countries recorded a consistent increase in their consumption of opioid analgesics from 1989 to 2009, when the consumption levels reached nearly 40,000 S-DDD per million inhabitants per day in the United States and more than 20,000 S-DDD in Canada, compared with 85 S-DDD per million inhabitants per day in Mexico.

54. In Europe, the consumption levels for opioid analgesics used for the treatment of pain also increased dramatically in the period 2000-2009. However, there continue to be large disparities in those consumption levels among European countries. The two countries with the highest consumption levels, Germany and Austria, reported consumption of about 20,000 and 16,000 S-DDD per million inhabitants per day, respectively. Five other countries reported consumption levels of more than 10,000 S-DDD and 21 countries reported levels between 1,000 and 10,000 S-DDD. In some countries in the region, mostly in Eastern and South-Eastern Europe, consumption levels increased only slightly or even decreased. Consumption in 3 countries (Belarus, Romania and the Russian Federation) amounted to fewer than 200 S-DDD per million inhabitants per day.[22] Four countries reported consumption levels below 100 S-DDD (Albania, Republic of Moldova, the former Yugoslav Republic of Macedonia and Ukraine).

Figure 4. North America: average consumption of opioid analgesics, 1997-1999 and 2007-2009

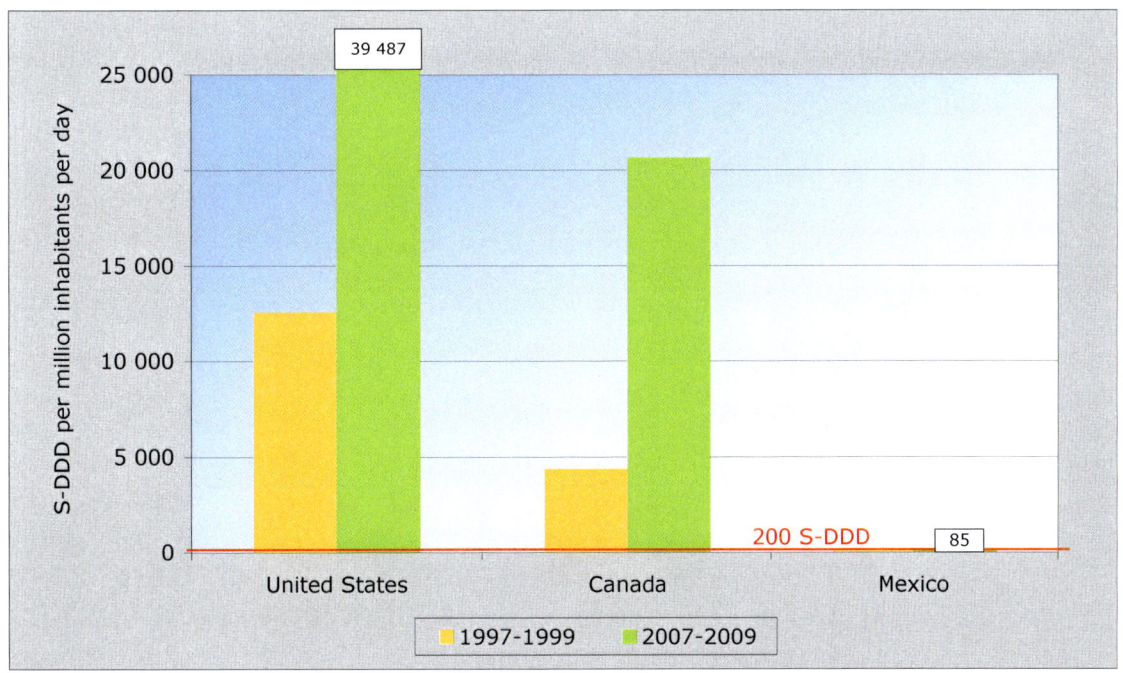

---

[22] Narcotic Drugs: Estimated World Requirements for 2011 — Statistics for 2009 (see footnote 16 above), table XIV.

REPORT ON THE AVAILABILITY OF INTERNATIONALLY CONTROLLED DRUGS

Figure 5a. Europe (countries with higher consumption): average consumption of opioid analgesics, 1997-1999 and 2007-2009

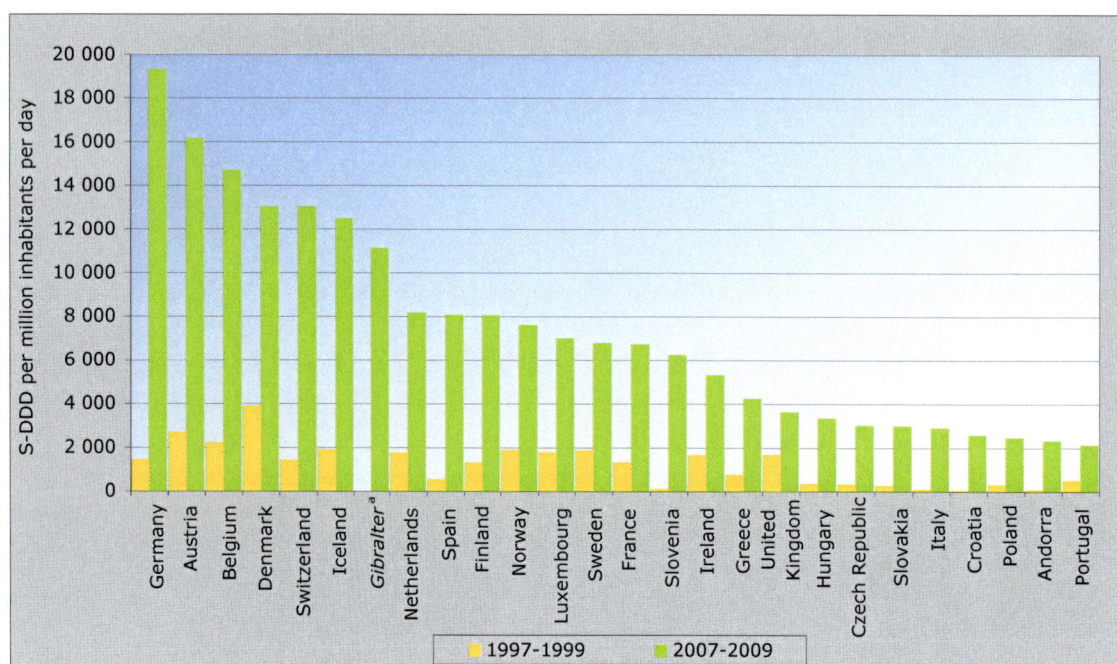

[a] Data not available, as the territory did not submit statistical forms for the three consecutive years 1997-1999.

Figure 5b. Europe (countries with lower consumption): average consumption of opioid analgesics, 1997-1999 and 2007-2009

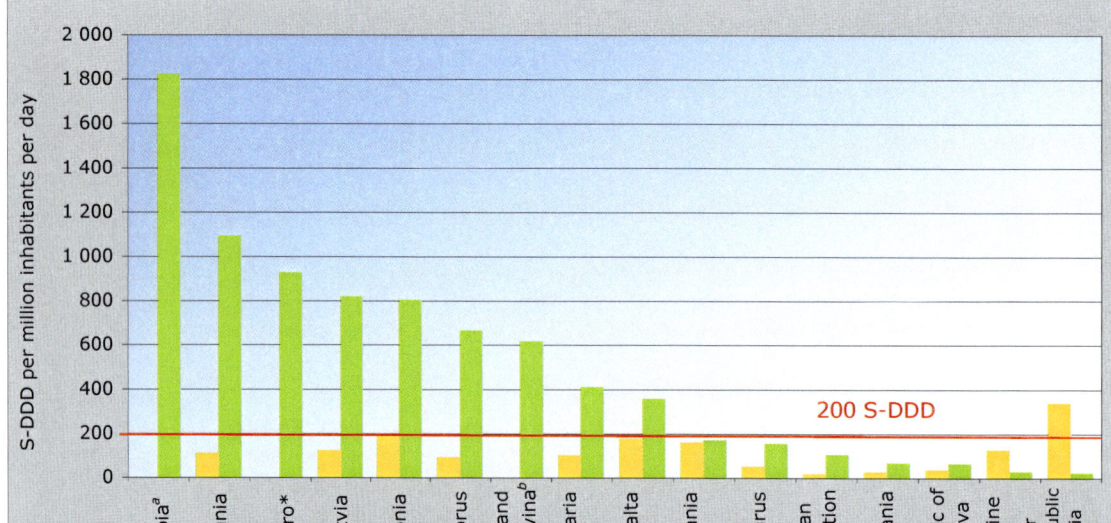

[a] Data for 1997-1999 not available, as the country was not admitted to membership in the United Nations until 2006.
[b] Data not available, as the country did not submit statistical forms for the three consecutive years 1997-1999.

AVAILABILITY OF MEDICINES CONTAINING INTERNATIONALLY CONTROLLED SUBSTANCES

55. Significant increases in the consumption of opioid analgesics also occurred in the period 2000-2009 in some countries in East and South-East Asia, West Asia, South America and Oceania. Despite those increases, the level of consumption of opioid analgesics remained relatively low in most countries in those regions.

56. In East and South-East Asia, the consumption levels for opioid analgesics in 65 per cent of the countries in the region amounted to fewer than 100 S-DDD per million inhabitants per day in the period 2007-2009. The highest levels of consumption were reported in Japan and the Republic of Korea, the two countries in the region that recorded the most dramatic increase in such consumption during the past decade (more than 1,000 S-DDD per million inhabitants per day). However, in most countries in the region, consumption levels for opioid analgesics increased only slightly. More than 80 per cent of the countries reported consumption levels below 200 S-DDD. In Cambodia, Indonesia, the Lao People's Democratic Republic and Myanmar, those consumption levels were below 10 S-DDD per million inhabitants per day. No consumption of opioid analgesics was reported by Timor Leste.

Figure 6. East and South-East Asia: average consumption of opioid analgesics, 1997-1999 and 2007-2009

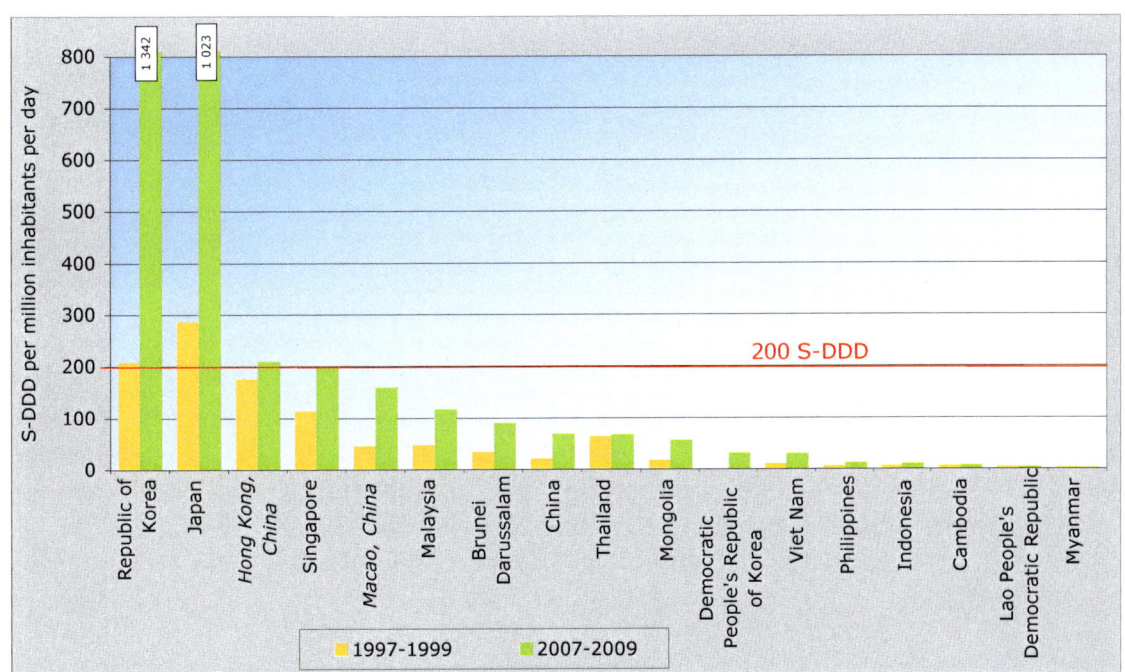

57. In West Asia, the consumption levels for opioid analgesics in more than 60 per cent of the countries in the region amounted to fewer than 100 S-DDD per million inhabitants per day in the period 2007-2009. Consumption levels in Israel have been substantially higher than in the other countries in the region and increased steadily over a 20-year period, reaching more than 3,000 S-DDD per million inhabitants per day in the period 2007-2009. The consumption levels for opioid analgesics used for the treatment of pain increased significantly in the period 2000-2009 in Bahrain and Turkey. Consumption increased but remained below 200 S-DDD in Jordan, Kuwait, Lebanon,

Qatar, Saudi Arabia and the United Arab Emirates. In Afghanistan, Iraq, Pakistan, Tajikistan, Uzbekistan and Yemen, consumption levels were below 10 S-DDD per million inhabitants per day in 2009.

Figure 7.   West Asia: average consumption of opioid analgesics, 1997-1999 and 2007-2009

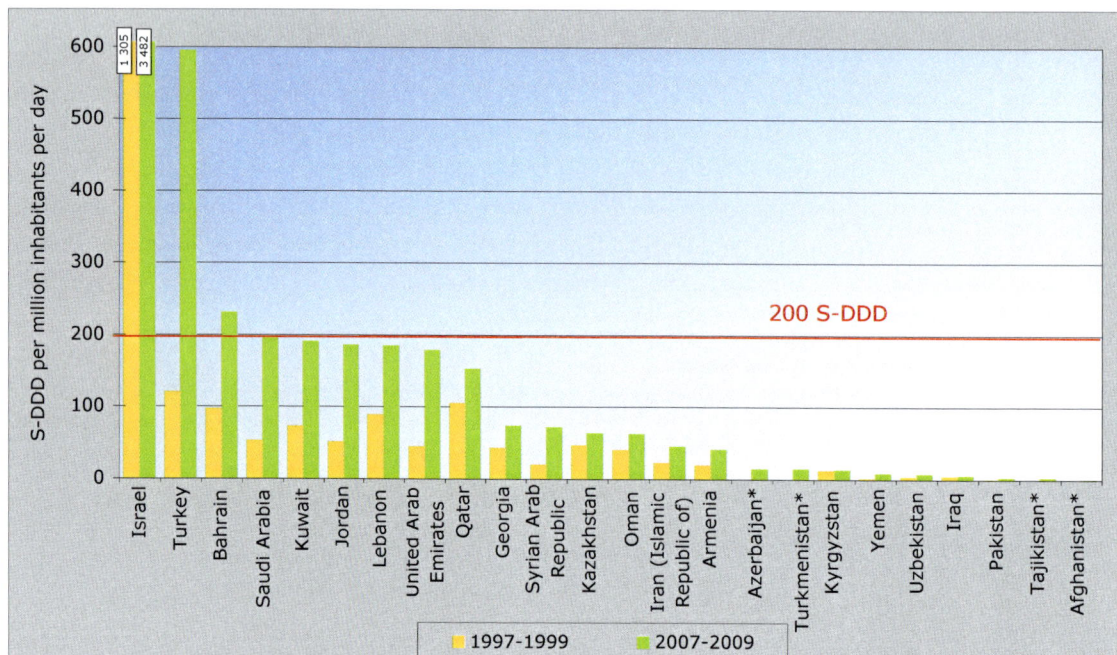

* Data not available, as the country did not submit statistical forms for the three consecutive years 1997-1999.

58. In South America, the consumption levels for opioid analgesics in more than 50 per cent of the countries in the region amounted to fewer than 100 S-DDD per million inhabitants per day in the period 2000-2009, although consumption levels in the region as a whole increased significantly. In about half of the countries in the region, consumption of opioid analgesics more than doubled during that period. The highest consumption level in the period 2007-2009 was reported by the Falkland Islands (Malvinas), with 4,283 S-DDD per million inhabitants per day. Argentina and Chile reported consumption levels of about 400 S-DDD per million inhabitants per day. Bolivia (Plurinational State of) and Guyana reported consumption of opioid analgesics to be no more than 10 S-DDD per million inhabitants per day.

59. In Oceania, the situation with regard to consumption levels in the different countries is sharply divided. Of 15 reporting countries, 6 (40 per cent) have consumption levels below 100 S-DDD per million inhabitants per day. On the other hand, 7 countries (47 per cent) reported consumption of more than 1,000 S-DDD. The consumption levels for opioid analgesics in Australia for the period 2007-2009 (more than 8,000 S-DDD) were substantially higher than in the other countries in the region. Despite significant increases in the consumption levels for opioid analgesics in the Marshall Islands, Nauru, Papua New Guinea, Samoa, Tonga and Vanuatu, consumption levels remained low (less than 100 S-DDD per million inhabitants per day).

Figure 8. South America: average consumption of opioid analgesics, 1997-1999 and 2007-2009

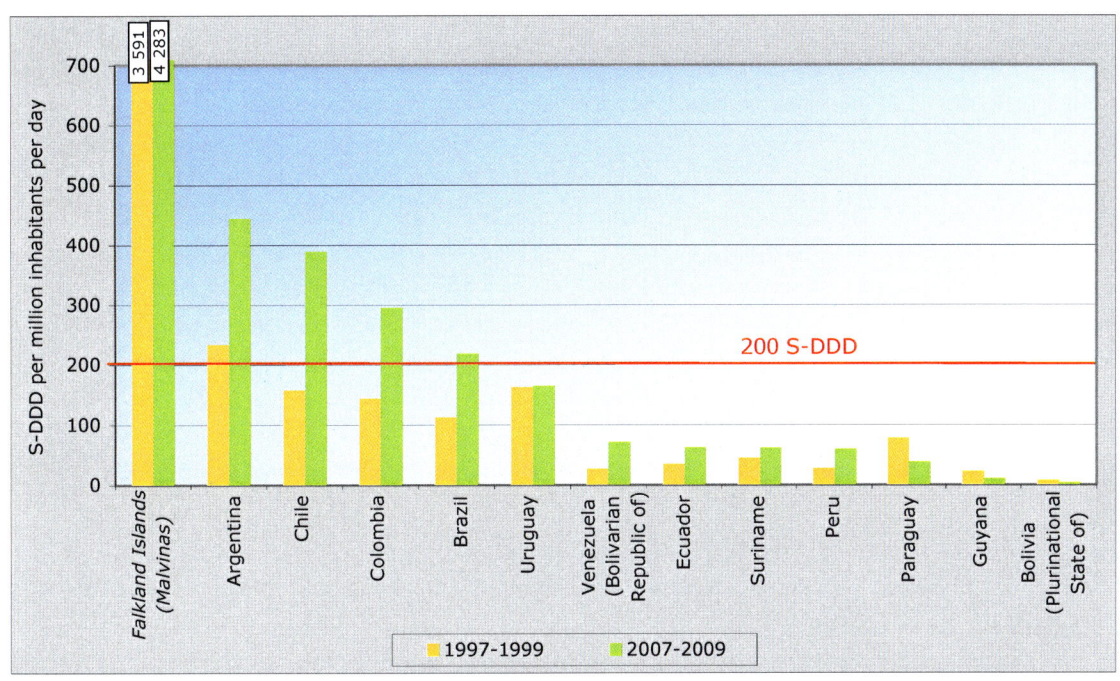

Figure 9. Oceania: average consumption of opioid analgesics, 1997-1999 and 2007-2009

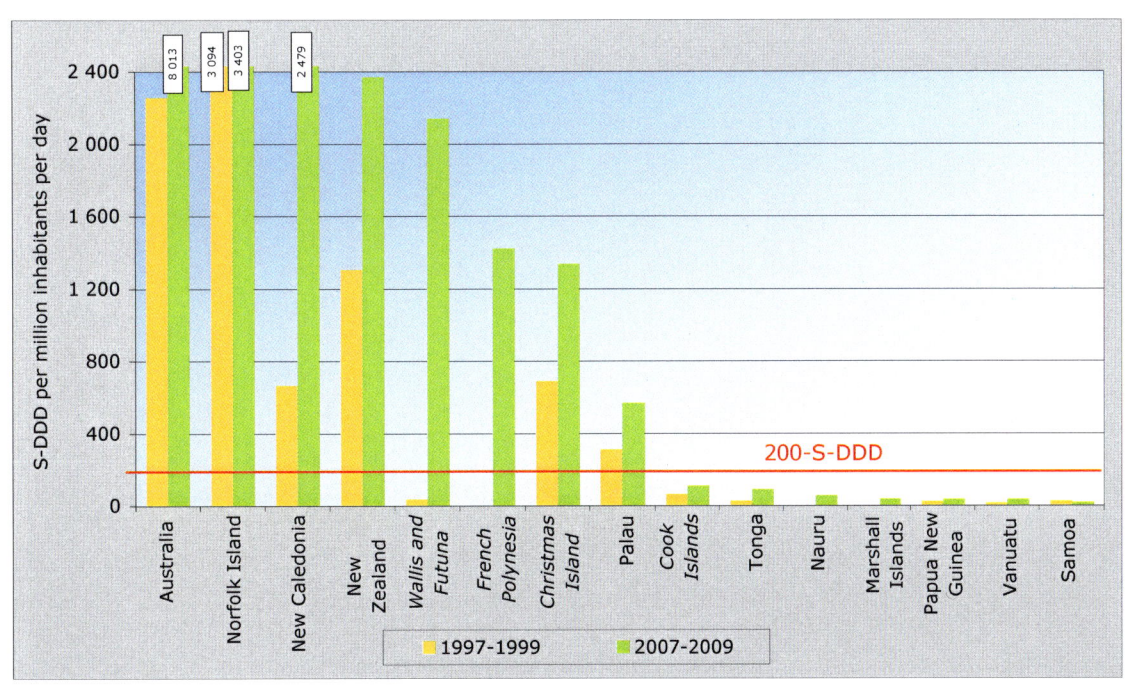

60. In contrast to the developments in the above-mentioned regions, consumption levels for opioid analgesics in Africa, Central America and the Caribbean and South Asia did not increase significantly in the period 2000-2009. Modest increases were recorded in a few countries in each of those three regions. As a result, in the vast majority of the countries in those regions consumption of opioid analgesics amounted to fewer than 100 S-DDD per million inhabitants per day, and in a large number of those countries less than 10 S-DDD or even zero.

61. Africa has continued to be the region with the lowest levels of consumption for opioid analgesics. Only one country reported consumption above 200 S-DDD per million inhabitants per day, and four others reported consumption of above 100 S-DDD. In nearly 90 per cent of the countries in the region, such consumption amounted to fewer than 100 S-DDD per million inhabitants per day, and nearly half of the countries in the region had levels below 5 S-DDD. Significant increases in consumption have been limited to a few countries, and it has decreased in several others. South Africa currently has the highest consumption level for opioid analgesics in the region, averaging 600 S-DDD per million inhabitants per day. In six countries in the region (Cameroon, Chad, Mali, Nigeria, Rwanda and United Republic of Tanzania), average consumption of opioid analgesics amounted to less than 1 S-DDD per million inhabitants per day. No consumption of opioid analgesics was reported by the Central African Republic, the Congo, Djibouti, Equatorial Guinea, the Gambia, Guinea, Guinea-Bissau, Liberia, Somalia or Swaziland.

Figure 10a. Africa (countries with higher consumption): average consumption of opioid analgesics, 1997-1999 and 2007-2009

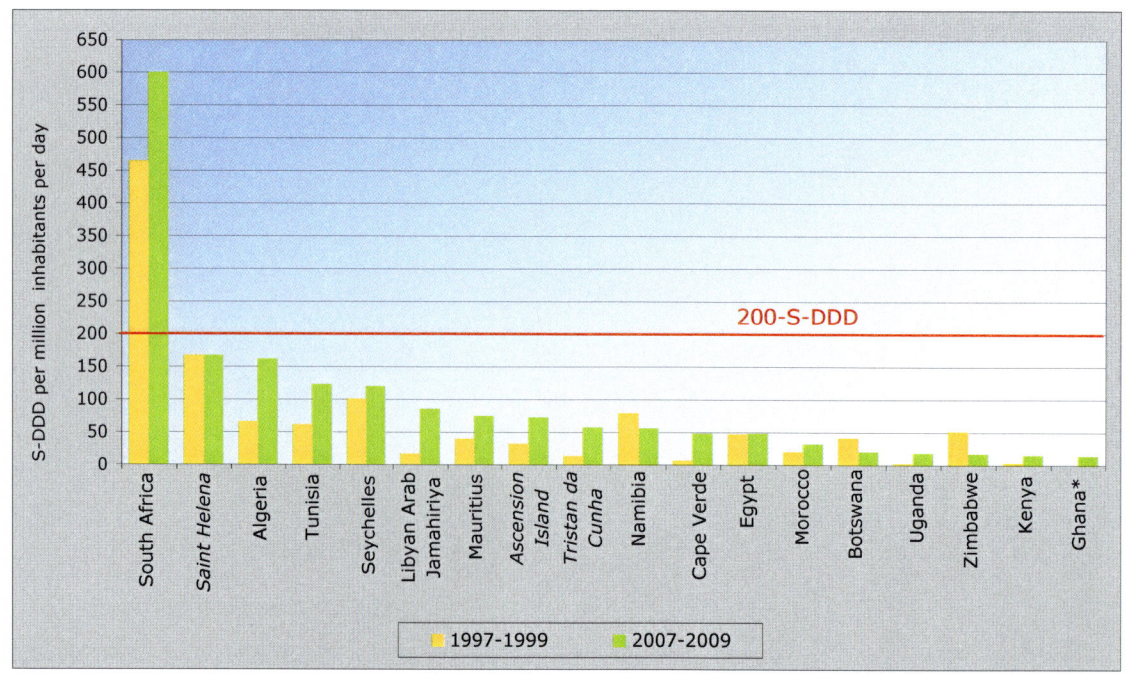

* Data not available, as the country did not submit statistical forms for the three consecutive years 1997-1999.

Figure 10b. Africa (countries with lower consumption): average consumption of opioid analgesics, 1997-1999 and 2007-2009

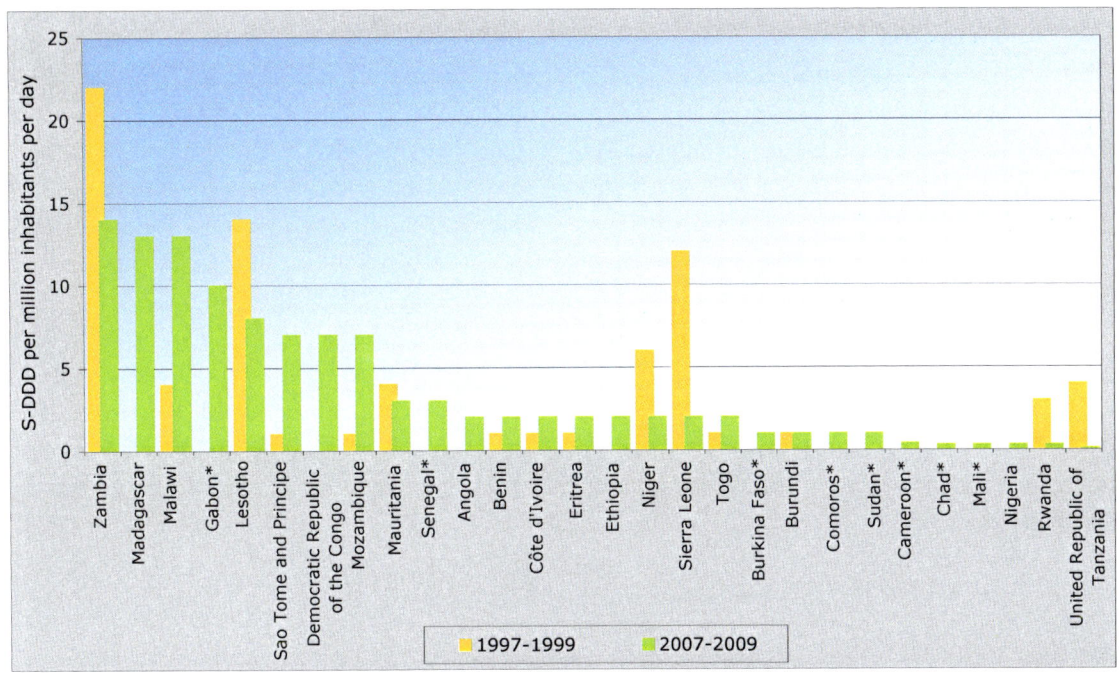

* Data not available, as the country did not submit statistical forms for the three consecutive years 1997-1999.

62. In Central America and the Caribbean, consumption levels for opioid analgesics remained relatively low in the period 1989-2009. More than half of the countries in the region reported levels of fewer than 100 S-DDD of opioid analgesics per million inhabitants per day in the period 2007-2009. Only the Cayman Islands and the Netherlands Antilles reported consumption above 1,000 S-DDD per million inhabitants per day. Haiti reported average consumption of 2 S-DDD per million inhabitants per day. No consumption of opioid analgesics was reported by Anguilla, Antigua and Barbuda, Aruba, Barbados, Belize, the British Virgin Islands, Honduras or Saint Kitts and Nevis.

63. All countries in South Asia reported very low consumption levels of opioid analgesics during the period 2007-2009. The highest consumption level was reported by Sri Lanka, with 26 S-DDD. Bhutan was the only other country with a consumption level above 20 S-DDD. Bangladesh and Nepal reported consumption of less than 10 S-DDD.

64. As indicated in the paragraphs above, there continue to be large disparities among countries in terms of the consumption of opioids. Opioid analgesics under international control continue not to be available in sufficient quantities to meet the medical requirements of the population in many countries throughout the world, including in several countries with very large populations, such as India and Nigeria. In some other countries, however, overprescribing and the availability of opioid analgesics in quantities greater than those required for sound medical treatment may lead to the diversion and abuse of those substances, which some countries are already experiencing.

REPORT ON THE AVAILABILITY OF INTERNATIONALLY CONTROLLED DRUGS

B. Opioids controlled under the 1971 Convention

65. Buprenorphine, lefetamine and pentazocine are the analgesics controlled under the 1971 Convention. The consumption of buprenorphine, an opioid analgesic in Schedule III of the 1971 Convention, accounted for over 99 per cent of global consumption of such analgesics in 2009. Calculated consumption of buprenorphine increased sharply in the period 1990-2009, although the information available is not accurate enough to allow the level of consumption to be calculated for each of the major manufacturing and consuming countries. Two decades ago, buprenorphine was used in only 12 countries, none of them in Africa or Oceania. In the period 2007-2009, buprenorphine was used in about 75 countries or territories, representing every region, or about 35 per cent of all countries and territories. That shift in the use of buprenorphine is attributable to its increasing use in higher-dosage forms for the treatment of pain and for substitution treatment. Australia, Belgium, France, Germany, Norway, the United Kingdom of Great Britain and Northern Ireland and the United States are the countries with the highest consumption levels for buprenorphine. Europe has consistently been the region with the highest levels of consumption.

Figure 11. Central America and the Caribbean: average consumption of opioid analgesics, 1997-1999 and 2007-2009

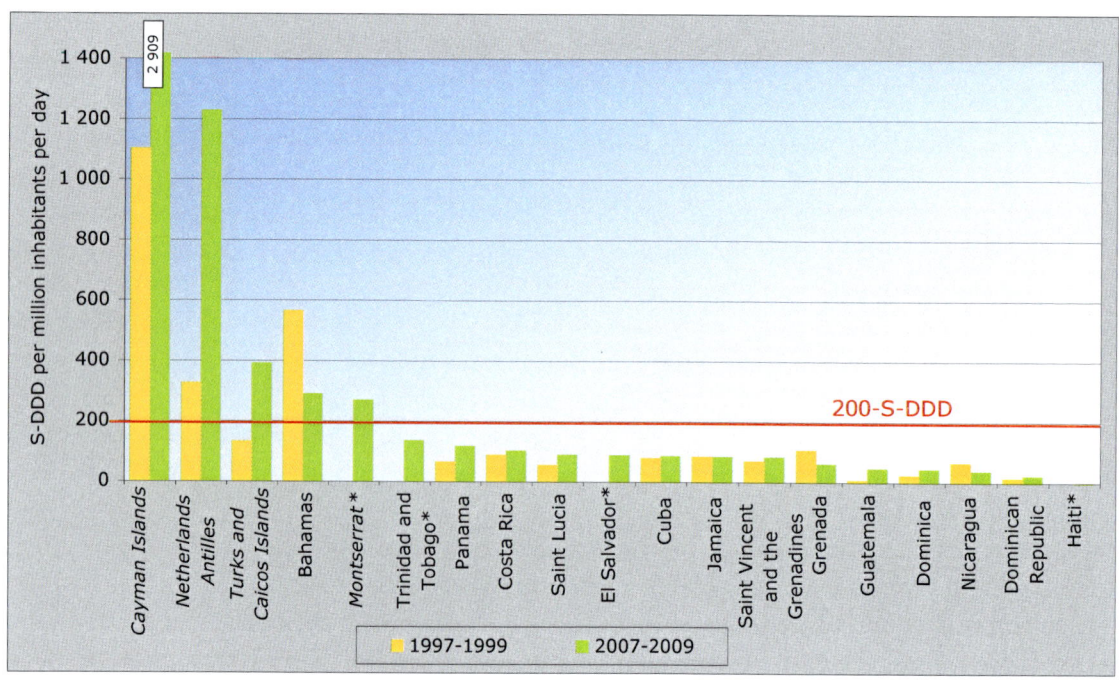

* Data not available, as the country or territory did not submit statistical forms for the three consecutive years 1997-1999.

Figure 12. South Asia: average consumption of opioid analgesics, 1997-1999 and 2007-2009

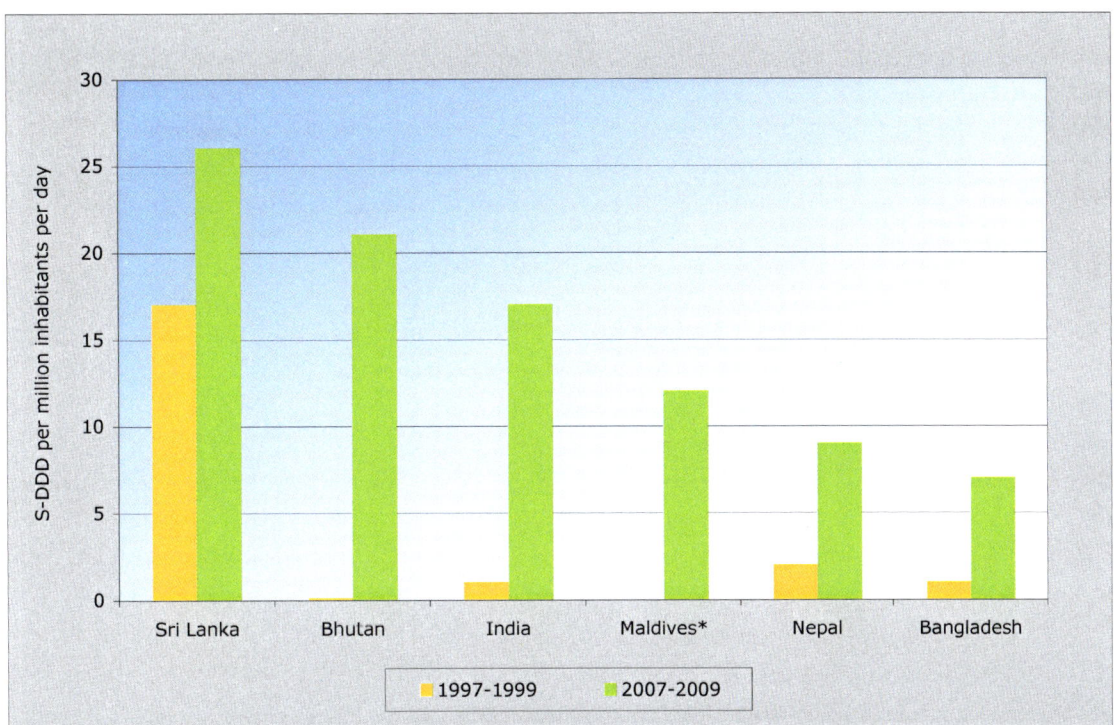

* Data not available, as the country did not provide consumption data for the three consecutive years 1997-1999.

66. From the information available, it is not possible to identify countries with problematic consumption patterns (consumption levels that are too low or too high), mainly because of the reporting problems mentioned above, but also because certain narcotic drugs (for example, any opioid analgesic for the treatment of pain and methadone for substitution treatment) might be used as a substitute for buprenorphine, and its availability should be reviewed in connection with the availability of those drugs. The diversion of buprenorphine from domestic distribution channels, above all from substitution treatment programmes, continues to occur.

67. Pentazocine is an opioid analgesic with properties and uses similar to those of morphine; it is listed in Schedule III of the 1971 Convention. In the period 2005-2009, global calculated consumption of pentazocine showed a slight increase. In contrast to the use of buprenorphine, pentazocine use is not spreading to other countries; the same 50 countries have been using pentazocine during the last decade, among which India, Pakistan and the United States together accounted for 80 per cent of the global total in the period 2007-2009.

C. Anti-epileptics

68. Clonazepam (a benzodiazepine), methylphenobarbital and phenobarbital are the anti-epileptics controlled under the 1971 Convention. All three of them are in Schedule IV of that Convention. In addition to being used for the treatment of epilepsy, they are used to induce sleep. From the data reported to the Board, it is not possible to determine the extent to which the substances are used to induce sleep and the extent to which they are used to treat epilepsy. The consumption of phenobarbital accounted for over 99 per cent of global consumption of anti-epileptics in 2009.

69. Calculated consumption of anti-epileptics increased in the period 1990-2009. In 1990, the use of those substances was reported in 120 countries throughout the world. Since then, their use has spread to virtually every country, and phenobarbital is one of the most widely used psychotropic substances. As is the case for all psychotropic substances, calculated consumption levels for anti-epileptics based on the data reported to the Board are very tentative, as some major manufacturers and importers submit inaccurate or inconsistent data. The countries with the highest consumption levels for anti-epileptics are Bulgaria, Latvia and Ukraine. Europe has consistently been the region with the highest consumption levels for those substances.

Figure 13. Selected countries: average consumption[a] of methylphenidate, 1997-1999 and 2007-2009

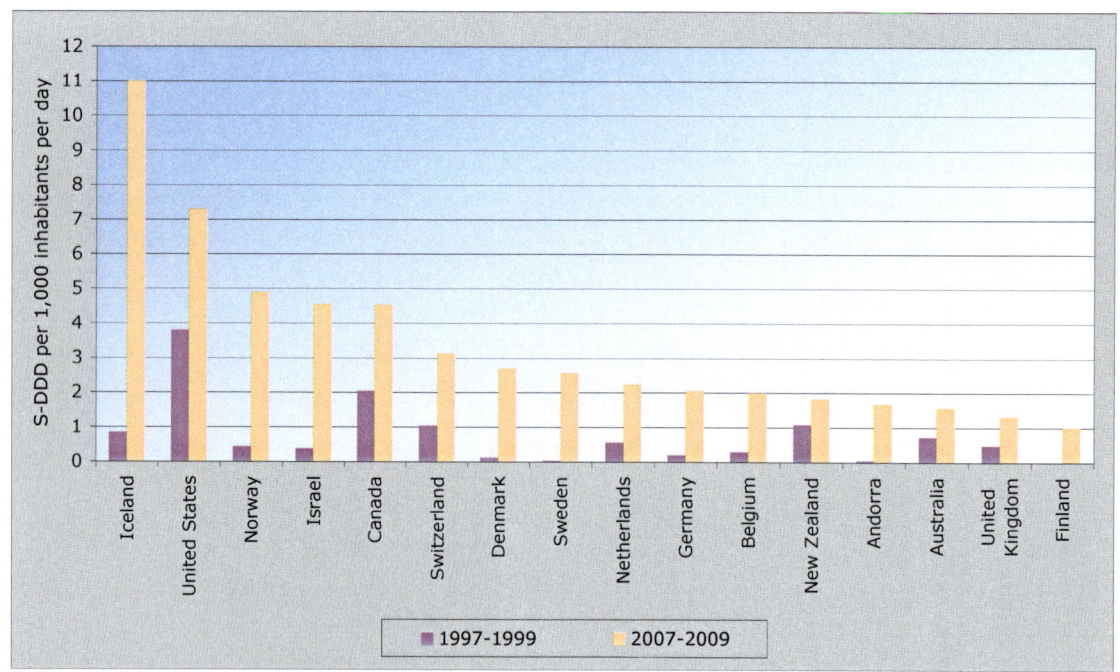

[a] Approximate consumption calculated by the Board.

70. In Benin, the consumption levels for anti-epileptics (7 S-DDD per million inhabitants per day in 2008) are much higher than the average for Africa, which could indicate excessive availability linked to non-implementation of the prescription requirements foreseen by the 1971 Convention, as well as the possibility of related diversion and abuse. The information available to the Board does not allow conclusions to be drawn as to whether the substances are available in all countries in sufficient quantities, in particular as anti-epileptics. Diverted phenobarbital is sometimes found on illicit markets, possibly because the substance is not available on licit markets in the quantities required. There have been enquiries from hospitals indicating that in some countries the quantities of phenobarbital imported for medical purposes are not sufficient.

D. Stimulants in Schedule II of the 1971 Convention that are used for the treatment of attention deficit disorder

71. Methylphenidate, amphetamine and dexamphetamine, substances in Schedule II of the 1971 Convention, are used mainly for the treatment of attention deficit disorder (ADD) and narcolepsy. For many years, the most extensive use of those substances for medical purposes has been in the Americas. In recent years, the highest levels of consumption for those stimulants have been observed in Canada, Israel, the United States and countries in northern Europe.

72. Methylphenidate is the most widely used stimulant in Schedule II of the 1971 Convention. Its manufacture and use continue to increase. In the period 2005-2009, global calculated consumption of methylphenidate increased by 30 per cent, reaching 40 tons, the majority of which was accounted for by the United States. In that country, the use of methylphenidate for the treatment of ADD continues to be promoted in advertisements directed at potential consumers, contrary to the provisions of the 1971 Convention. The use of methylphenidate for the treatment of ADD has been growing in many other countries as well, although the use of the substance continues to be much greater in the United States than in all the other countries combined. Countries other than the United States together accounted for less than 20 per cent of global calculated consumption of methylphenidate in 2000; however, that proportion gradually increased to 30 per cent by 2009.

73. During the period 2007-2009, about 100 countries and territories reported the use of methylphenidate and about 70 reported the use of amphetamines. Stimulants in Schedule II of the 1971 Convention appear not to be available in about 50 per cent of all countries and territories. Since 2007, Iceland, followed by the United States, has been the country with the highest calculated per capita consumption of methylphenidate. Figure 13 shows the countries with consumption rates of methylphenidate above 1 S-DDD per thousand inhabitants per day, ranked by their calculated consumption levels.

74. As previously noted by the Board, the diversion and abuse of stimulants in Schedule II of the 1971 Convention take place in countries with very high levels of consumption of those substances. The Board reiterates its request to all Governments to ensure that the control measures foreseen in the 1971 Convention are fully applied to stimulants in Schedule II.

E. Stimulants in Schedule IV of the 1971 Convention that are used as anorectics

75. The stimulants in Schedule IV of the 1971 Convention are used mainly as anorectics. The most frequently used stimulant in Schedule IV is phentermine, followed by fenproporex, amfepramone and mazindol.

Figure 14. All regions: average consumption[a] of central nervous system stimulants in Schedule IV, 1997-1999 and 2007-2009

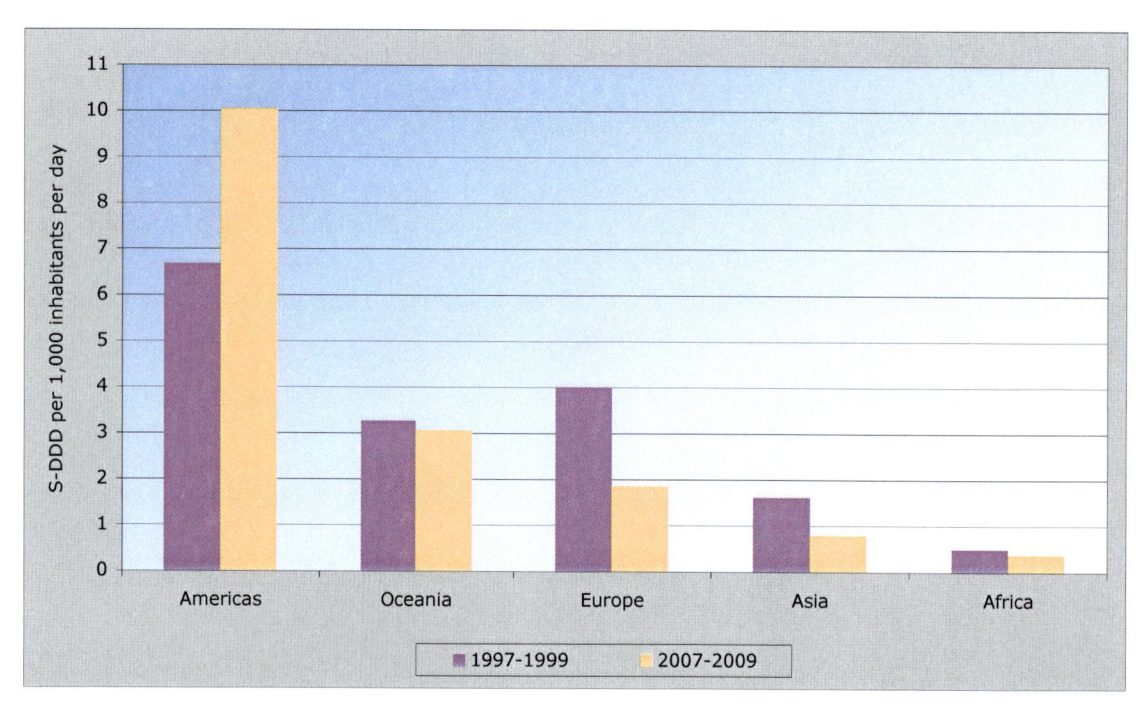

[a] Approximate consumption calculated by the Board.

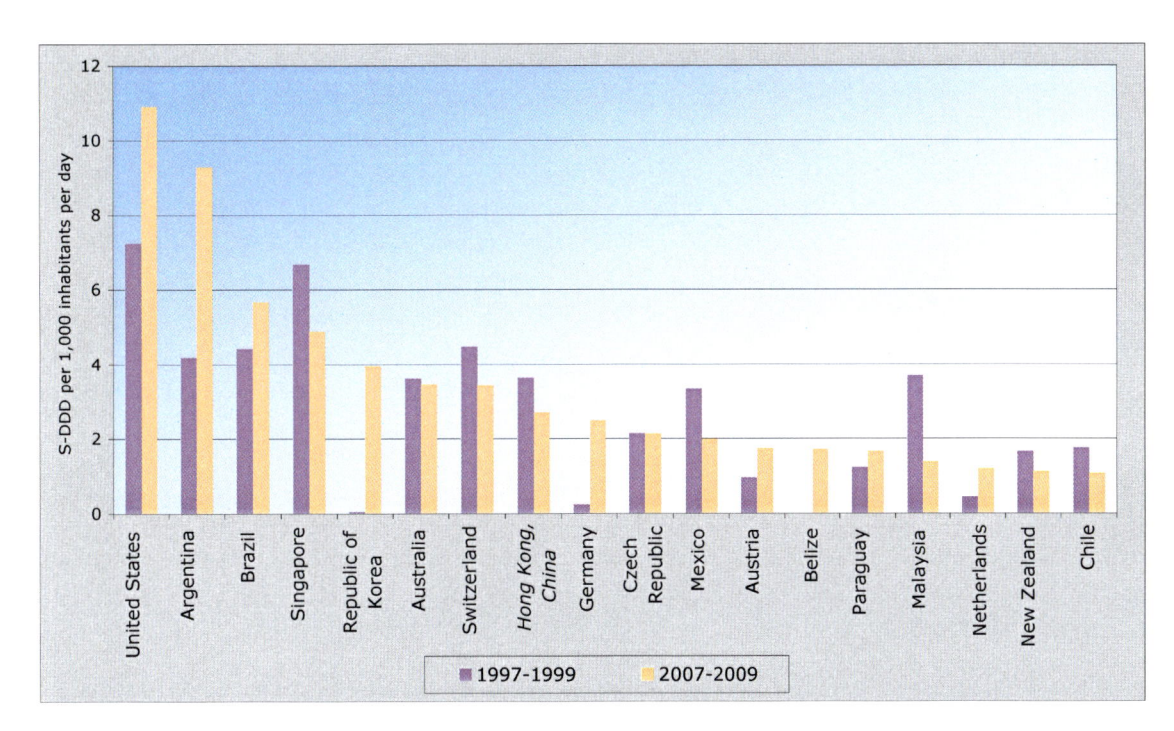

AVAILABILITY OF MEDICINES CONTAINING INTERNATIONALLY CONTROLLED SUBSTANCES

Figure 15. Selected countries and territories: average consumption[a] of central nervous system stimulants in Schedule IV, 1997-1999 and 2007-2009

[a] Approximate consumption calculated by the Board.

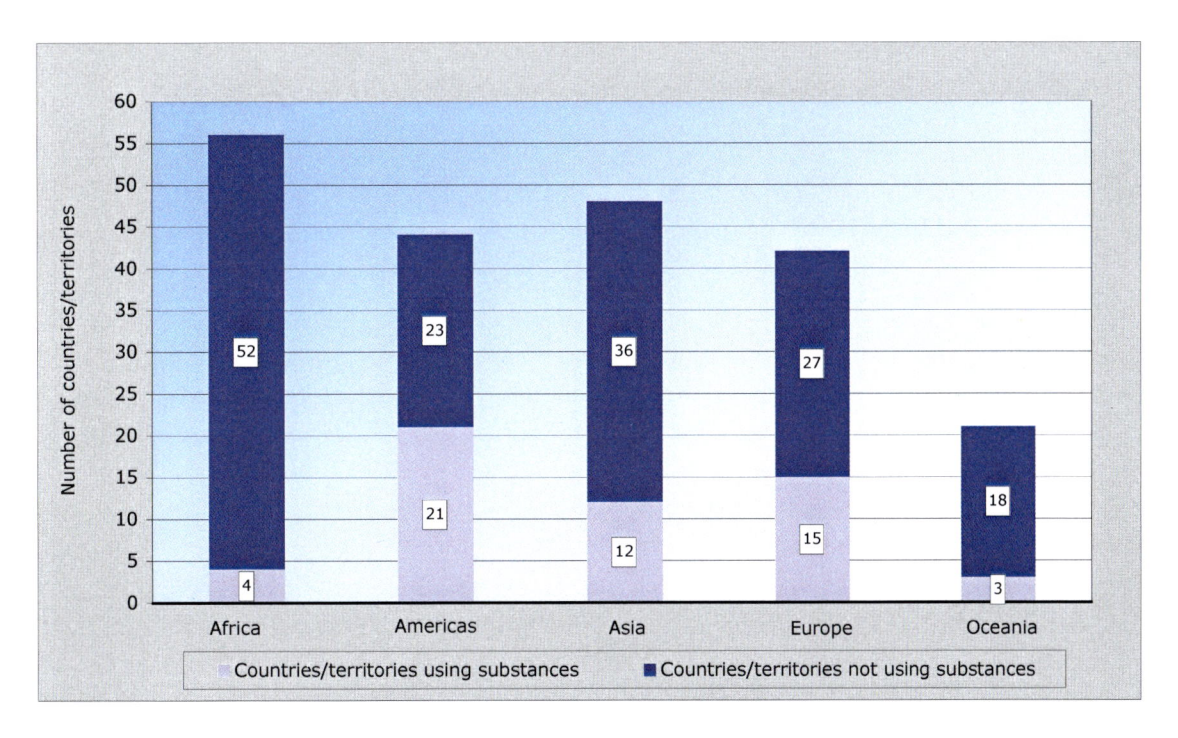

Figure 16. All regions: number of countries and territories using central nervous system stimulants in Schedule IV, 2007-2009

76. The highest calculated consumption levels for stimulants in Schedule IV of the 1971 Convention have traditionally been recorded in countries in the Americas, in particular Argentina, Brazil and the United States. In the period 2007-2009, average calculated consumption in the Americas continued to increase, and the United States remained the country with the world's highest calculated per capita consumption levels for those stimulants. Until 2006, Brazil had similar levels of consumption. Between 2006 and 2009, Brazil succeeded in reducing per capita consumption of those stimulants by two thirds by strictly enforcing the prescription requirement and taking action against members of the medical profession who were found to have acted in an unprofessional manner. The share of global calculated consumption of stimulants in Schedule IV (expressed in S-DDD) accounted for by the United States increased from 58 per cent in 2008 to 71 per cent in 2009. The declining demand for stimulants has been noted by the industry: in 2009 global manufacture of this group of stimulants decreased by 25 per cent from the level of previous years, mainly because of a drop in the manufacture of fenproporex in Brazil.

77. About 75 countries and territories report regular use of stimulants included in Schedule IV of the 1971 Convention. Figure 15 reflects the fact that consumption levels of those stimulants vary greatly between countries and regions, whereas figure 16 shows for each region the number of countries and territories that reported such use. In about 60 per cent of all the countries and territories, those stimulants appear not to be available; their availability is particularly limited in Africa, the island countries of Oceania and much of Asia.

78. In a number of countries, high prescription levels for stimulants in Schedule IV have led to the diversion and abuse of those stimulants. The Board encourages Governments to remain vigilant and identify consumption levels that are inappropriate and/or not required for sound medical practice and to take steps to fully apply the control measures foreseen in the 1971 Convention.

F. Benzodiazepines

79. For benzodiazepines, global calculated consumption shows a slight increase in the last decade. During that period, practically all countries and territories that reported to the Board manufactured or traded in benzodiazepines in quantities of more than 1 kg at least once. Among anxiolytics, alprazolam and diazepam are the most used substances, whereas triazolam was the most consumed sedative-hypnotic. Reporting obligations for substances included in Schedules III and IV, such as benzodiazepines, are less stringent than for Schedule II substances. Calculated consumption levels for these types of substances are therefore more approximate than for Schedule II substances.[23]

---

[23] Figures 17 to 28 provide information on global and regional developments in consumption levels of benzodiazepines over the last 10 years. Owing to the significant differences in consumption levels, the scales used in the figures vary.

AVAILABILITY OF MEDICINES CONTAINING INTERNATIONALLY CONTROLLED SUBSTANCES

Benzodiazepine-type anxiolytics

80. As can be seen in figure 17, consumption levels of benzodiazepine-type anxiolytics are highest in countries in Europe, reflecting the fact that benzodiazepines tend to be prescribed frequently for the elderly. As reflected in figures 19 to 22, consumption levels of benzodiazepine-type anxiolytics in countries outside of Europe in the period 2007-2009 tended to be lower than 20 S-DDD per thousand inhabitants per day, although there were a few exceptions.

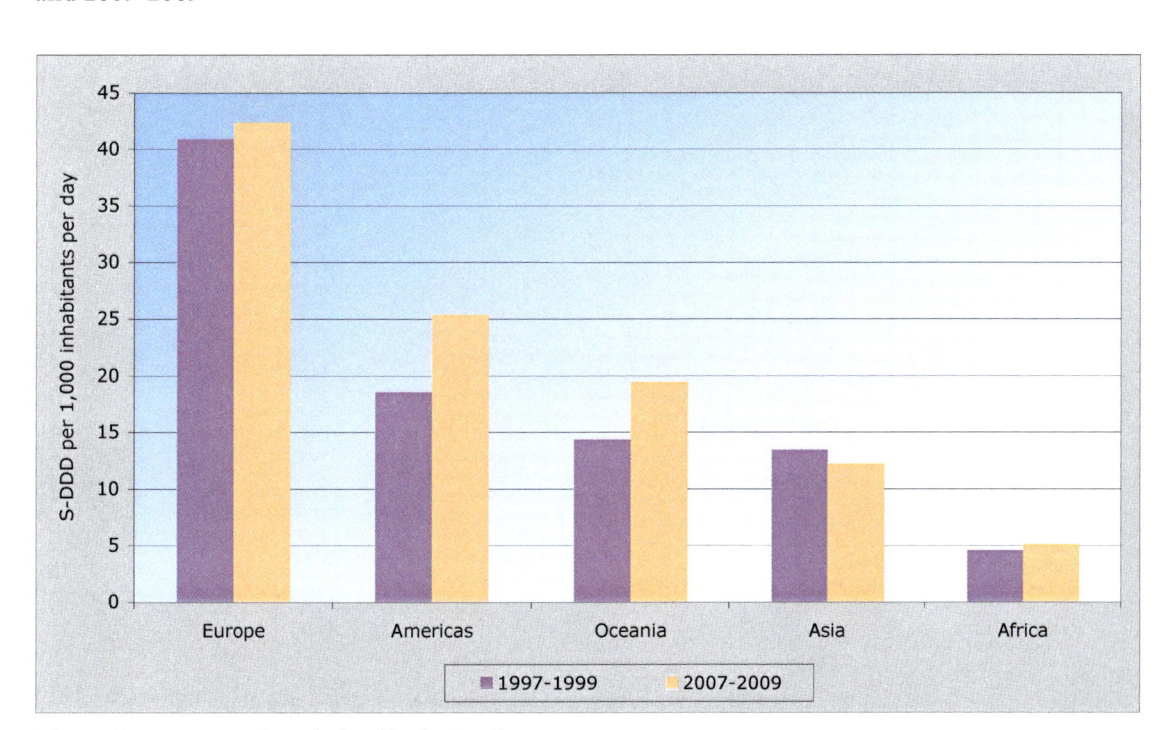

Figure 17. All regions: average consumption[a] of benzodiazepines (anxiolytics), 1997-1999 and 2007-2009

[a] Approximate consumption calculated by the Board.

81. Consumption of anxiolytics in many countries in Europe during the last decade increased from an already high level. Between 2007 and 2009, in 12 countries (about 27 per cent of the region), calculated average consumption levels exceeded 40 S-DDD per thousand inhabitants, and in another 14 countries (31 per cent) those levels were between 20 and 40 S-DDD per thousand inhabitants. Countries in Western and South-Eastern Europe have the highest consumption levels in the region.

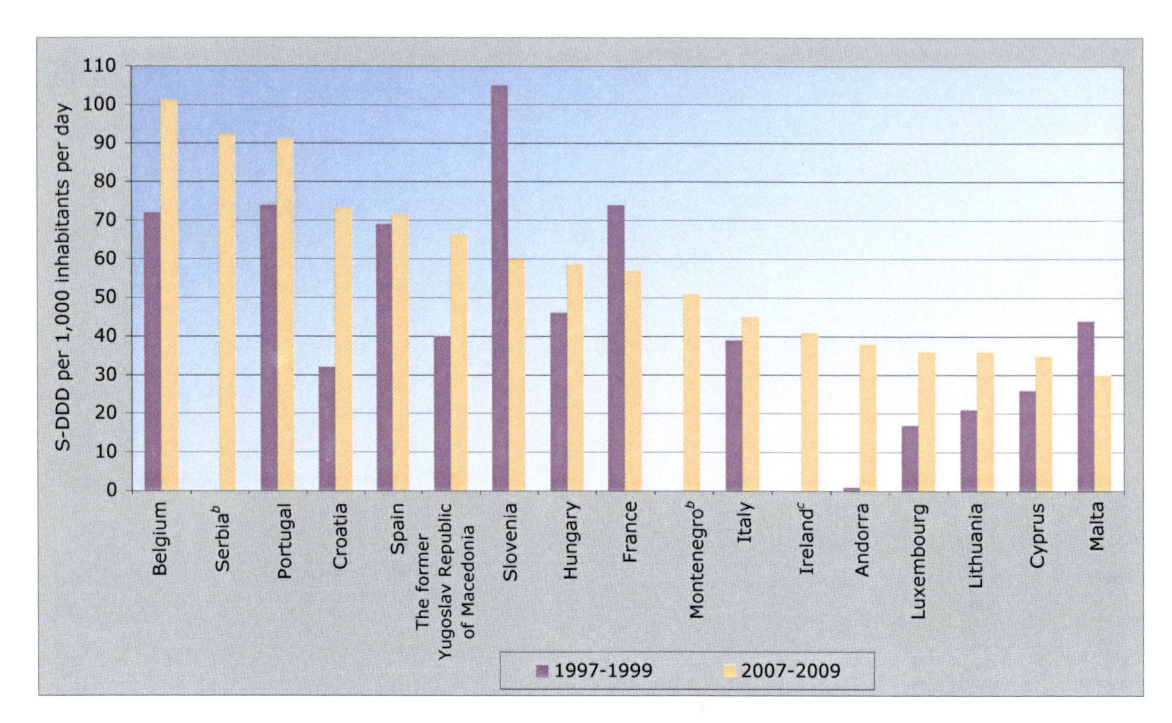

Figure 18. Europe (selected countries): average consumption[a] of benzodiazepines (anxiolytics), 1997-1999 and 2007-2009

[a] Approximate consumption calculated by the Board.
[b] Countries constituted after 1999, therefore, no data are available for the period 1997-1999.
[c] Data received do not allow calculation of approximate consumption for the period 1997-1999.

82. In Africa, Ghana showed the highest average calculated consumption of anxiolytics (16 S-DDD per thousand inhabitants) in the period 2007-2009. For six countries (Algeria, Benin, Cape Verde, Democratic Republic of the Congo, Tunisia and South Africa), consumption was between 5 and 10 S-DDD per thousand inhabitants per day. Eight countries, as shown in figure 19, had consumption levels between 1 and 5 S-DDD per thousand inhabitants per day, whereas in all other countries and territories (73 per cent of the region) less than 1 S-DDD per thousand inhabitants per day was consumed.

83. In Asia, seven countries (Islamic Republic of Iran, Iraq, Israel, Japan, Jordan, Pakistan and Republic of Korea) (15 per cent of the countries and territories) showed an average calculated consumption level of anxiolytics higher than 10 S-DDD per thousand inhabitants per day between 2007 and 2009, whereas in four countries and two territories (Lebanon, Sri Lanka, Syrian Arab Republic, Thailand, Hong Kong, China and Macao, China) consumption levels between 5 and 10 S-DDD per thousand inhabitants per day were observed. Ten countries (Bahrain, Cambodia, China, Georgia, India, Kuwait, Republic of Korea, Singapore, Turkey and Yemen) consumed between 2 and 5 S-DDD per thousand inhabitants per day. The remaining 44 per cent of the countries and territories in Asia consumed less than 2 S-DDD per thousand inhabitants per day.

AVAILABILITY OF MEDICINES CONTAINING INTERNATIONALLY CONTROLLED SUBSTANCES

Figure 19. Africa (selected countries): average consumption[a] of benzodiazepines (anxiolytics), 1997-1999 and 2007-2009

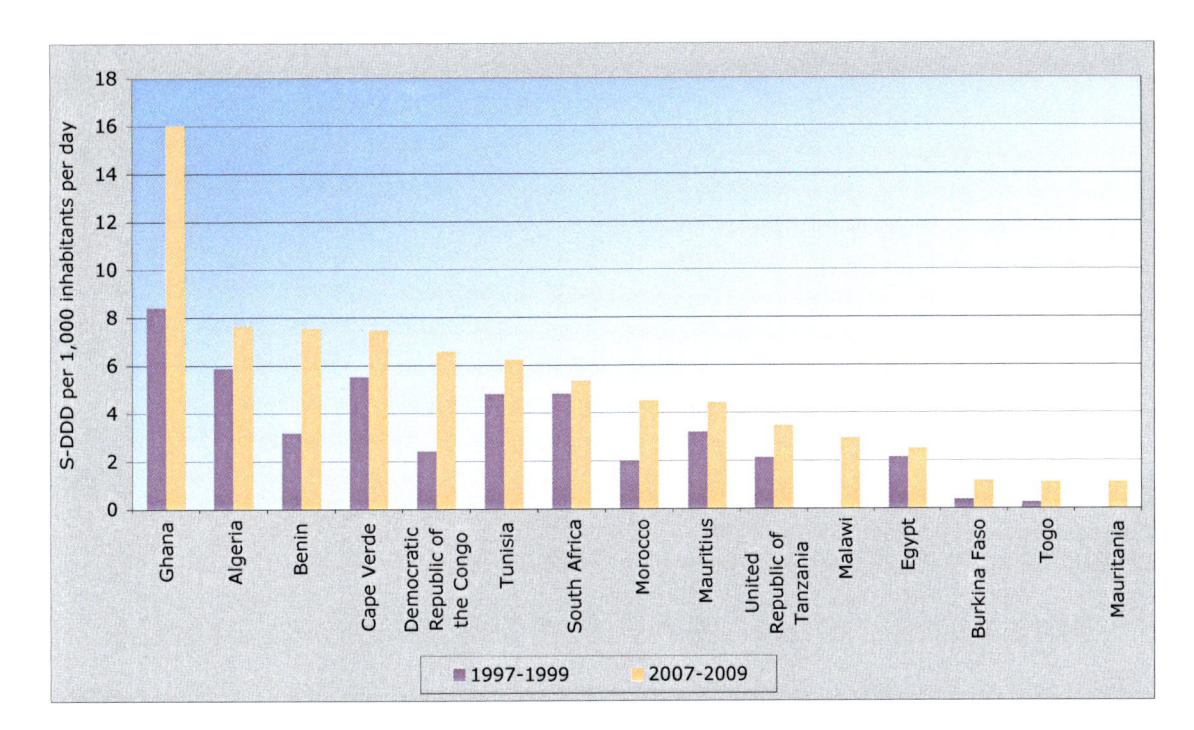

[a] Approximate consumption calculated by the Board.

Figure 20. Asia (selected countries and territories): average consumption[a] of benzodiazepines (anxiolytics), 1997-1999 and 2007-2009

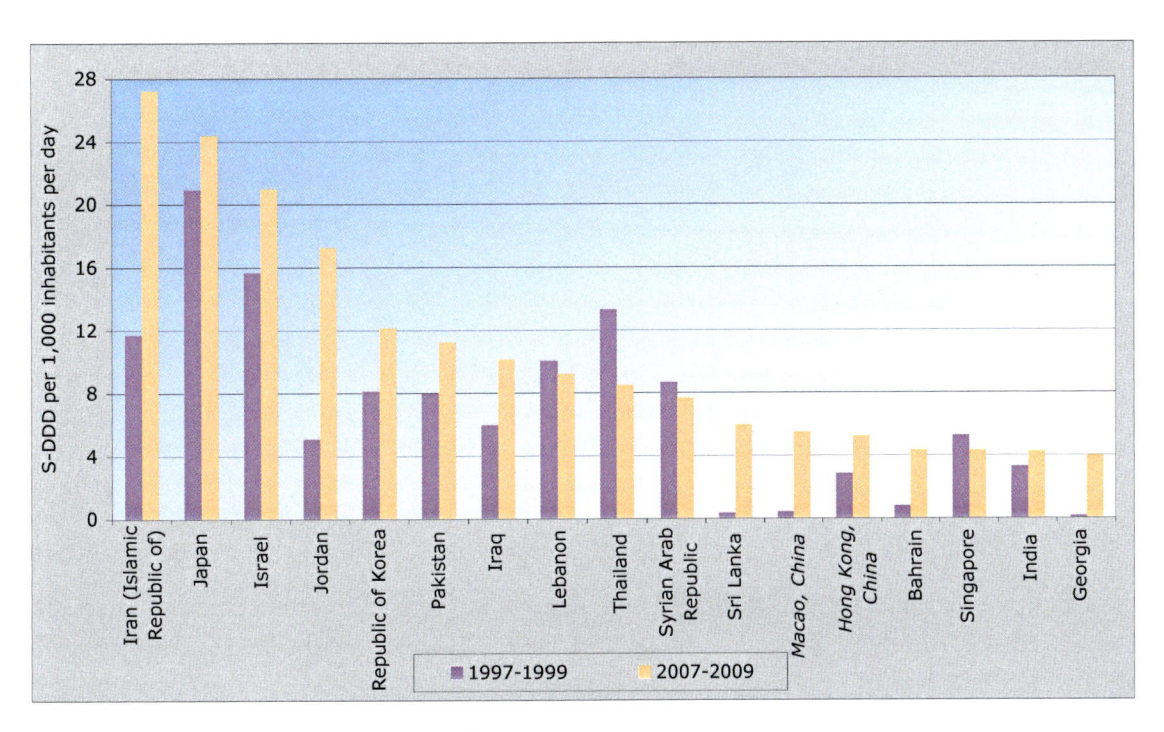

[a] Approximate consumption calculated by the Board.

REPORT ON THE AVAILABILITY OF INTERNATIONALLY CONTROLLED DRUGS

84. In Oceania, two countries and two territories (Australia, New Zealand, French Polynesia and New Caledonia) consumed on average more than 5 S-DDD of anxiolytics per thousand inhabitants per day in the period 2007-2009. All other countries and territories consumed considerably less.

85. In the Americas there are significant disparities in consumption levels of anxiolytics, as shown in figure 22. Apart from Argentina, the United States and Uruguay, which consumed on average more than 20 S-DDD of anxiolytics per thousand inhabitants per day between 2007 and 2009, six countries (Brazil, Canada, Chile, Cuba, Guyana and Paraguay) consumed between 10 and 20 S-DDD per thousand inhabitants per day, and five countries consumed between 5 and 10 S-DDD per thousand inhabitants per day. The great majority of countries and territories in the region (70 per cent) consumed less than 5 S-DDD of anxiolytics per thousand inhabitants per day. The high consumption levels observed for Argentina and Uruguay, which might indicate excessive availability and non-implementation of the prescription requirements foreseen by the 1971 Convention, may be related to the very high consumption of anorectics in the subregion.

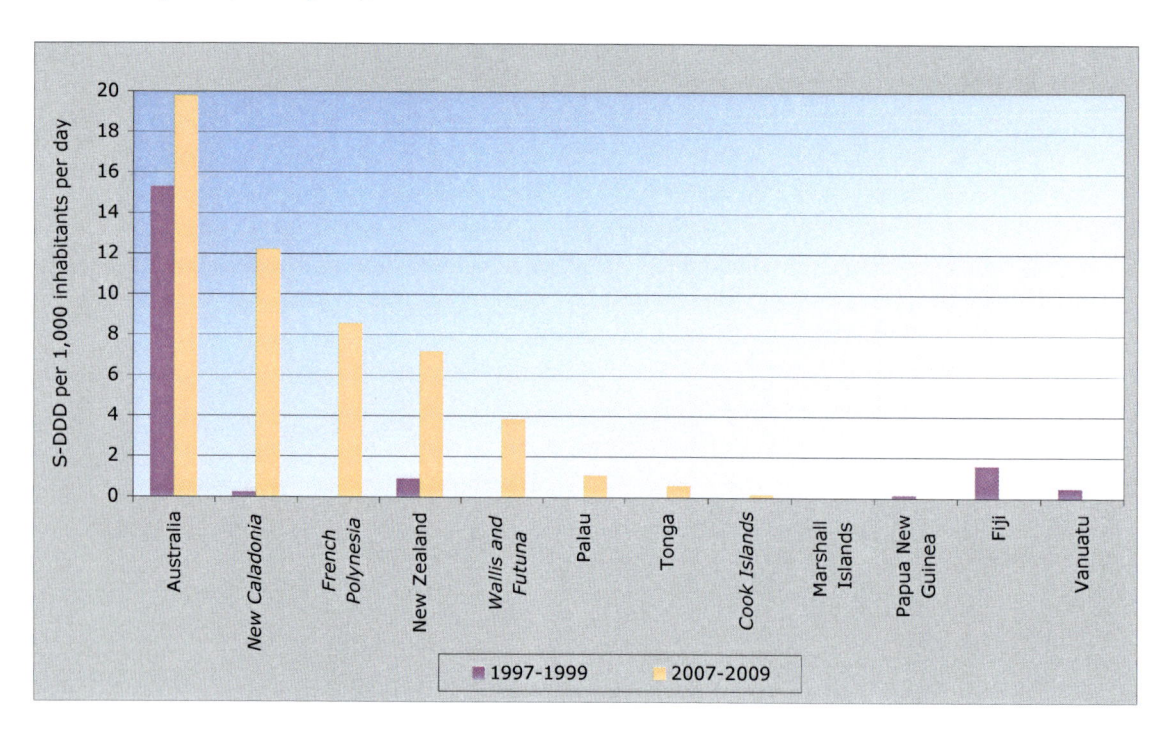

Figure 21. Oceania (selected countries and territories): average consumption[a] of benzodiazepines (anxiolytics), 1997-1999 and 2007-2009

[a] Approximate consumption calculated by the Board.

Benzodiazepine-type sedative-hypnotics

86. Among all the regions, calculated consumption levels of benzodiazepine-type sedative-hypnotics were consistently highest in Europe, as shown in figure 23. However, consumption of benzodiazepine-type sedative-hypnotics decreased in many countries in Europe and elsewhere in much more pronounced fashion than in the case of anxiolytics, from the levels observed a decade before, reflecting changes in the types of benzodiazepines that were prescribed in medical practice.

AVAILABILITY OF MEDICINES CONTAINING INTERNATIONALLY CONTROLLED SUBSTANCES

Figure 22. Americas (selected countries and territories): average consumption[a] of benzodiazepines (anxiolytics), 1997-1999 and 2007-2009

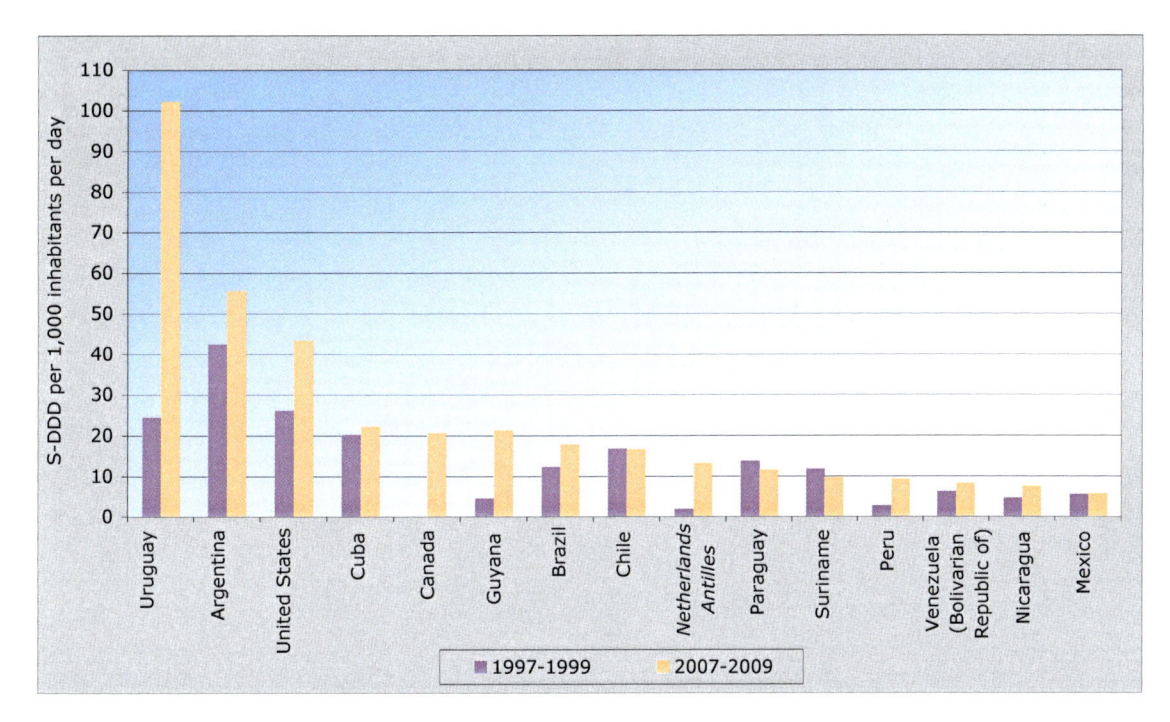

[a] Approximate consumption calculated by the Board.

Figure 23. All regions: average consumption[a] of benzodiazepines (sedative-hypnotics), 1997-1999 and 2007-2009

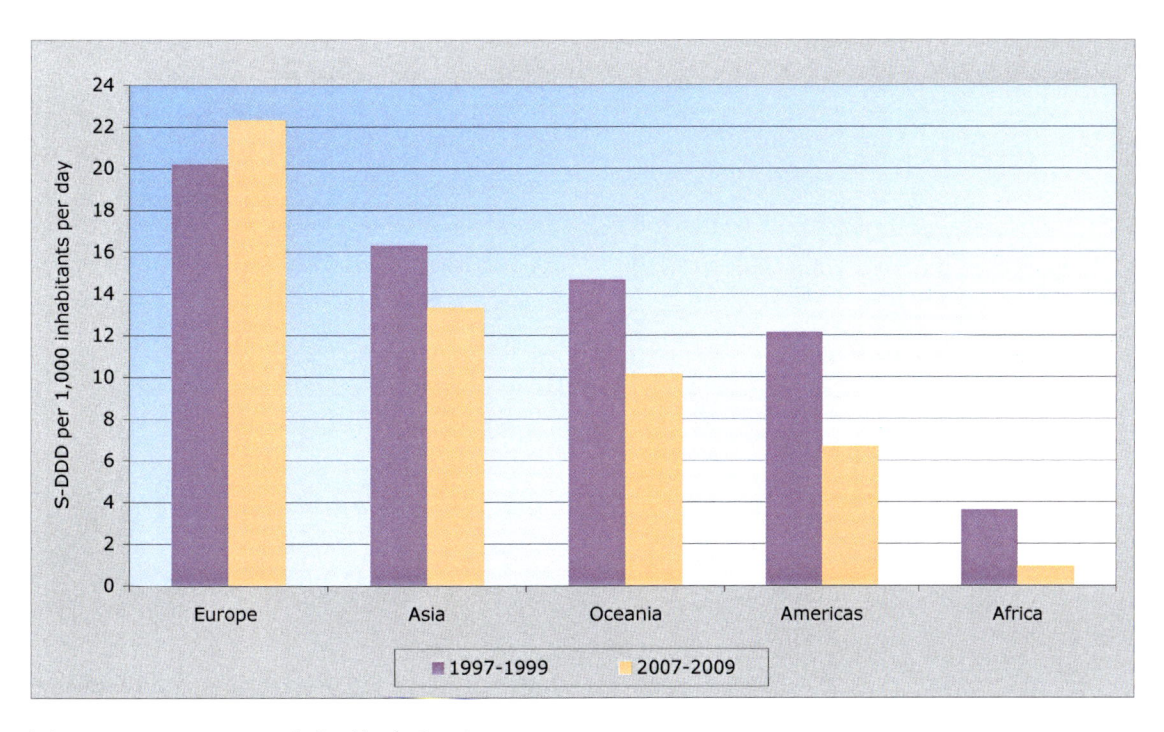

[a] Approximate consumption calculated by the Board.

87. In Europe, as shown in figure 24, in the period 2007-2009 average consumption levels of benzodiazepine-type sedative-hypnotics exceeded 10 S-DDD per thousand inhabitants in 13 countries (about 30 per cent of the region), and in another 8 countries (Andorra, Croatia, Greece, Ireland, Malta, Norway, Serbia and United Kingdom, accounting together for 18 per cent of the region) the corresponding consumption levels exceeded 5 S-DDD per thousand inhabitants. Countries in Western Europe showed the highest consumption levels in the region of this group of benzodiazepines.

88. In Africa, during the period 2007-2009 only Mauritius and South Africa showed an average calculated consumption of sedative-hypnotics higher than 1 S-DDD per thousand inhabitants. For five other countries (Cape Verde, Libyan Arab Jamahiriya, Namibia, Nigeria and Seychelles), consumption was between 0.1 and 1 S-DDD per thousand inhabitants per day. In five countries (Angola, Chad, Côte d'Ivoire, Ghana and Zambia) consumption levels were between 0.03 and 0.1 S-DDD per thousand inhabitants per day, whereas in all other countries and territories (82 per cent of the region) less than 0.03 S-DDD per thousand inhabitants per day was consumed.

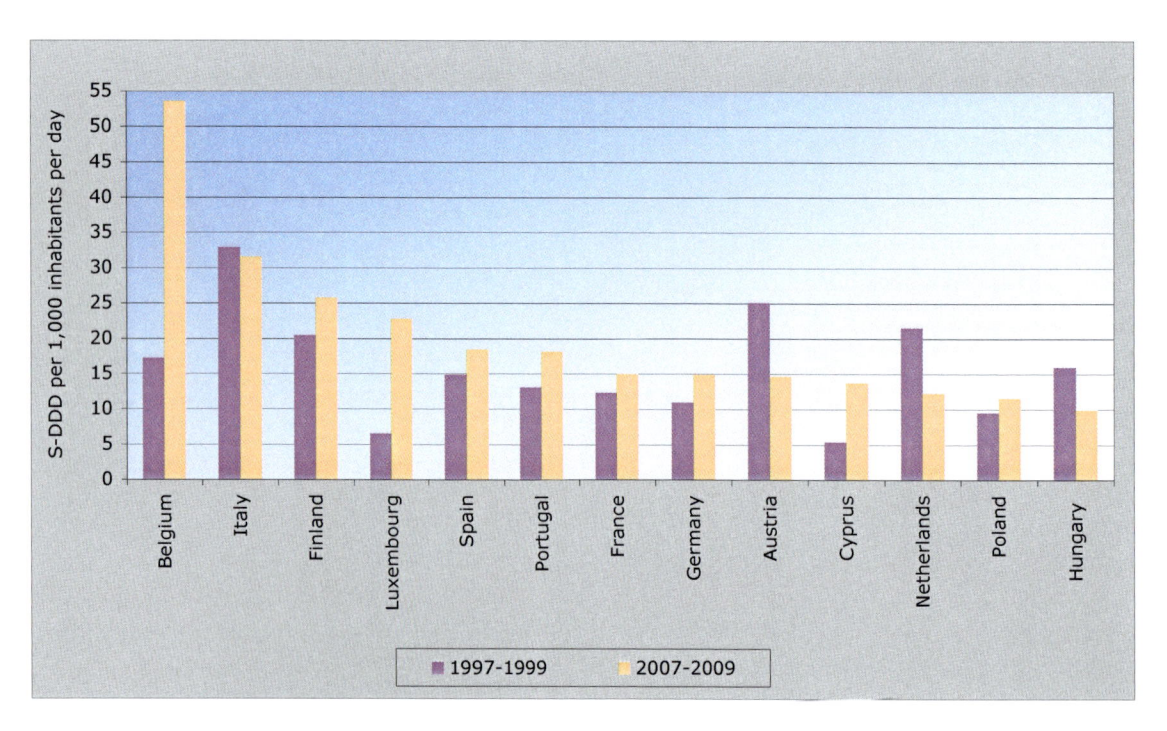

Figure 24. Europe (selected countries): average consumption[a] of benzodiazepines (sedative-hypnotics), 1997-1999 and 2007-2009

[a] Approximate consumption calculated by the Board.

Figure 25.   Africa (selected countries): average consumption[a] of benzodiazepines (sedative-hypnotics), 1997-1999 and 2007-2009

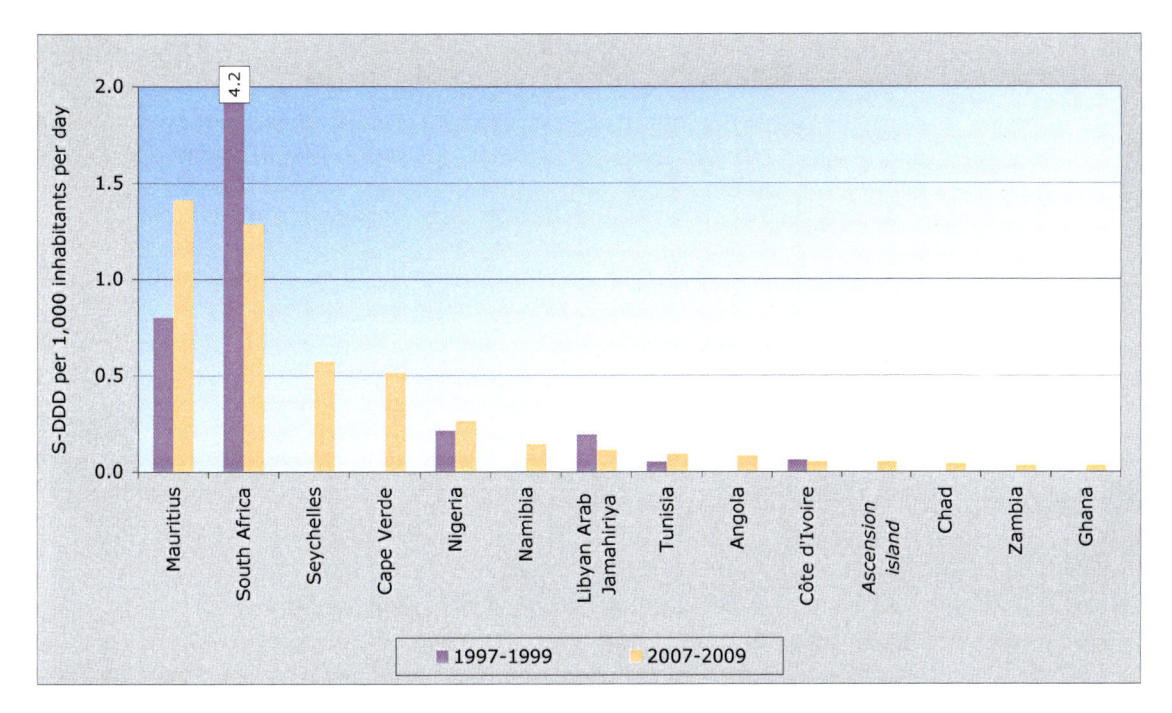

[a] Approximate consumption calculated by the Board.

Figure 26.   Asia (selected countries and territories): average consumption[a] of benzodiazepines (sedative-hypnotics), 1997-1999 and 2007-2009

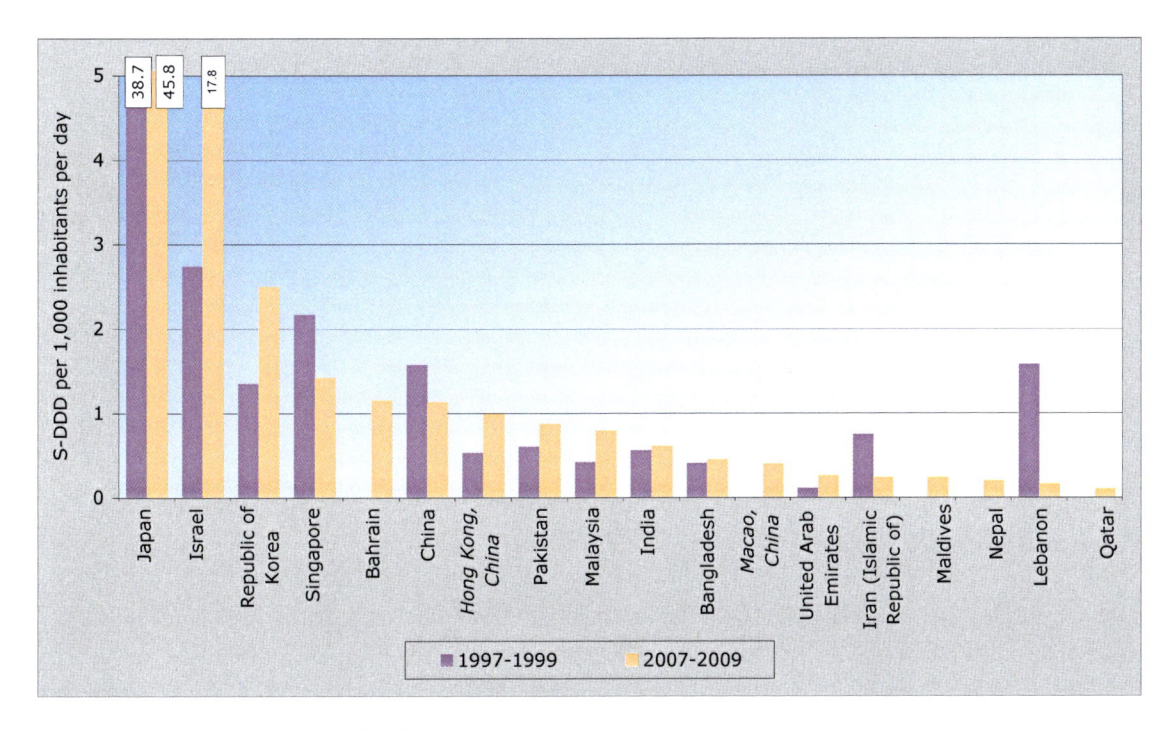

[a] Approximate consumption calculated by the Board.

89. In Asia, consumption levels of benzodiazepine sedative-hypnotics tend to be very low, except in Israel and Japan, which are the two countries in Asia with the largest populations of elderly people. The high consumption levels observed in Japan might also reflect inappropriate prescribing patterns and associated abuse. In the period 2007-2009, apart from Israel and Japan, four countries (Bahrain, China, Republic of Korea and Singapore) had consumption levels of more than 1 S-DDD of this group of benzodiazepines per thousand inhabitants per day, whereas the majority of countries and territories in the region (88 per cent) had levels of less than 1 S-DDD per thousand inhabitants per day.

90. In Oceania, in the period 2007-2009, only Australia and New Zealand had an average calculated consumption level of benzodiazepine-type sedative-hypnotics above 1 S-DDD per thousand inhabitants per day. Six other countries and territories had consumption levels of at least 0.01 S-DDD of this group of benzodiazepines per thousand inhabitants per day, as shown in figure 27. Although Fiji, the Marshall Islands, Papua New Guinea and Vanuatu imported and used benzodiazepine-type sedative-hypnotics, their calculated consumption levels were less than 0.01 S-DDD per thousand inhabitants per day.

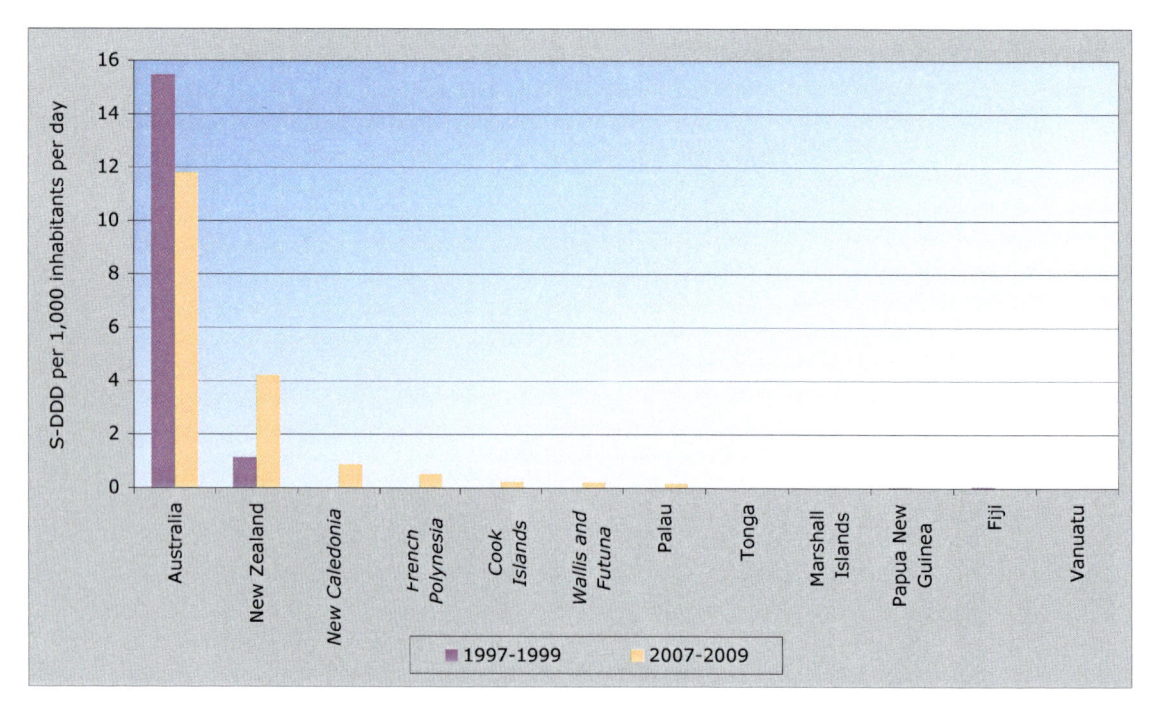

Figure 27. Oceania (selected countries and territories): average consumption[a] of benzodiazepines (sedative-hypnotics), 1997-1999 and 2007-2009

[a] Approximate consumption calculated by the Board.

91. In the Americas, in the period 2007-2009, Cuba and Uruguay had consumption levels averaging more than 10 S-DDD of benzodiazepine-type sedative-hypnotics per thousand inhabitants per day. Three countries (Canada, Paraguay and United States) had levels between 2 and 10 S-DDD per thousand inhabitants per day, and five countries and one territory (Argentina, Brazil, Chile, Panama,

Venezuela (Bolivarian Republic of) and Netherlands Antilles) had levels between 1 and 2 S-DDD per thousand inhabitants per day. The great majority of countries and territories in the region (80 per cent) had consumption levels of less than 1 S-DDD of benzodiazepine-type sedative-hypnotics per thousand inhabitants per day.

Figure 28. Americas (selected countries and territories): average consumption[a] of benzodiazepines, 1997-1999 and 2007-2009

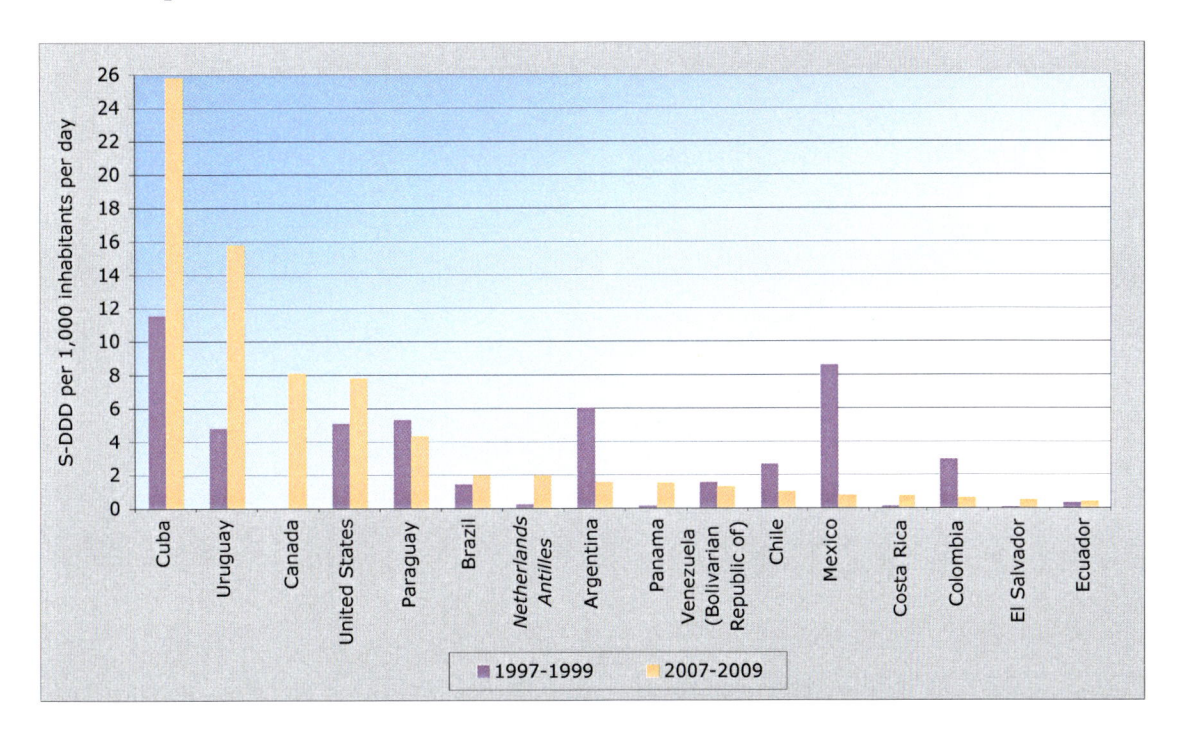

[a] Approximate consumption calculated by the Board.

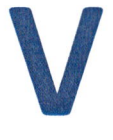

V. Achieving a balance between ensuring availability of internationally controlled substances for medical and scientific purposes and preventing their diversion and abuse

92. As affirmed in Commission on Narcotic Drugs resolution 53/4, on promoting adequate availability of internationally controlled licit drugs for medical and scientific purposes while preventing their diversion and abuse, the balance between adequate availability of these drugs and prevention of their diversion and abuse is at the core of the international drug control conventions. While in the absence of indicators of appropriate use it is at present not possible to determine what appropriate consumption levels would be in individual countries, let alone at the global level, it is possible to identify consumption levels that appear to be much too low or disproportionately high.

93. In the case of countries with nil or practically nil consumption levels, such indicators for adequate levels are not required, as there can be no doubt as to the inadequacy of availability. The Board considers all levels of consumption of narcotic drugs below 200 S-DDD per million inhabitants per day inadequate. However, this does not imply that levels above 200 S-DDD can be considered adequate as the determination of whether availability of internationally controlled substances required for treatment is sufficient depends on the specific morbidity data.

94. It may be of help to compare consumption levels between countries with similar levels of socio-economic development to determine whether a country's per capita consumption of certain drugs is in line with the levels prevalent in comparable countries. However, this method has two shortcomings. Low levels of consumption of internationally controlled substances are prevalent in certain regions. The fact that the majority of countries in a region record the same inadequately low levels of consumption does not make those levels adequate, but only indicates that most of the countries in the region face the same problem. On the other hand, disproportionately high levels of consumption of certain substances in a number of countries with comparable levels of socio-economic development do not make these consumption levels adequate. They could also indicate that prescription levels in all of those countries may be too high, and there could be a variety of reasons for this.

95. At present, therefore, circumstantial indicators are used to support other indicators of whether consumption levels are too low or too high. Reports on untreated patients and on difficulties in obtaining required medications indicate serious impediments to availability. Reports on diversion of internationally controlled substances from domestic distribution channels, on large-scale smuggling of such substances, on trafficking and on significant abuse might indicate availability of internationally controlled substances above levels required for sound medical practice.

A. Impediments to availability of opioid analgesics

96. The level of consumption of opioid analgesics in a country is generally correlated with its level of socio-economic development. There are a variety of factors determining why specific countries are found to have the highest levels of consumption of opioid analgesics in their region, including good reporting to and cooperation with the Board.

97. The Board has on a number of occasions drawn the attention of Governments to the causes of limited availability of opioids under international control. The causes include regulatory, attitudinal, knowledge-related, economic and procurement-related problems that adversely affect availability. In a recent survey conducted by the Board[24] on impediments to the availability of opioids for medical needs,[25] a majority of Governments reported that attitude- and knowledge-related impediments — namely, addiction-related concerns among health-care professionals and patients and insufficient training for health-care professionals — continued to be the main factors contributing to the underuse of opioids. Unduly restrictive laws and burdensome regulations were also commonly perceived as playing a significant role in limiting the availability of opioids. A smaller number of Governments reported that difficulties involving distribution and supply and the high cost of opioids were major obstacles to making opioids adequately available. The most important impediments listed by countries were concerns about addiction, reluctance to prescribe or stock and insufficient training for professionals. The ranking of importance of the various impediments as indicated by countries responding to the survey is shown in figure 29.

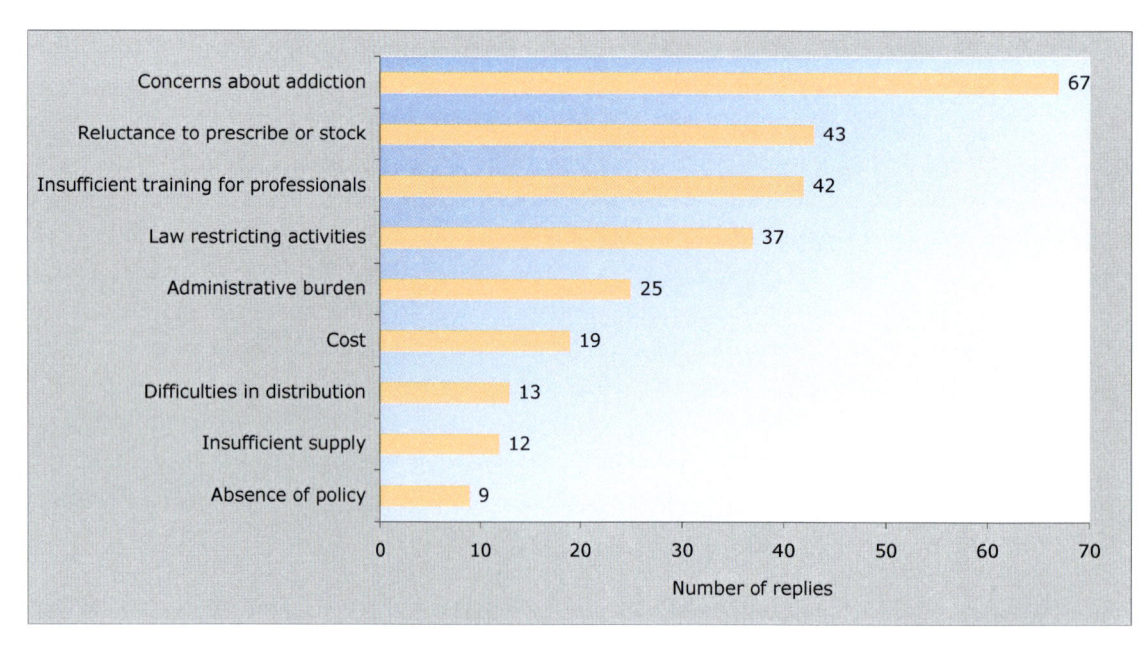

Figure 29. Main factors affecting the availability of opioids for medical needs

Factor	Number of replies
Concerns about addiction	67
Reluctance to prescribe or stock	43
Insufficient training for professionals	42
Law restricting activities	37
Administrative burden	25
Cost	19
Difficulties in distribution	13
Insufficient supply	12
Absence of policy	9

Note: The results shown in the figure are based on replies submitted by countries and territories in response to a specific multiple-choice question. They could choose one or more responses.

---

[24] The survey was carried out by means of the questionnaire on which figure 29 is based.
[25] Report of the International Narcotics Control Board on Follow-up to the Twentieth Special Session of the General Assembly (United Nations publication, Sales No. E.09.XI.7).

98. In many countries with low consumption levels for opioids, the availability of opioids is influenced by a combination of regulatory, knowledge-related and economic factors. Those factors are clearly not independent of one another; for example, it may be more difficult to bring about regulatory reforms in a country where concerns about drug addiction are pervasive among policymakers and health-care professionals. Overcoming those impediments therefore requires a multifaceted approach and the participation of a broad range of stakeholders from the relevant governmental regulatory bodies, health-care professionals and non-governmental organizations active in the field of health care.

99. France has successfully developed and implemented a multifaceted programme to ensure the adequate availability of opioid analgesics for the treatment of pain. Over the past decade, per capita consumption of opioid analgesics used in the treatment of moderate and severe pain has increased more than fivefold in France, making it one of the countries with apparently adequate and appropriate levels of consumption of opioid analgesics under international control.

100. After it was recognized that in France the level of consumption of analgesics was too low and pain was not being adequately treated in the health-care system, legislative and policy changes were introduced to promote the implementation of successive national action plans to combat pain, starting in 1989. Ensuring that health-care professionals are adequately educated about the treatment of pain has been an important element of each action plan. To that end, modules on pain treatment and palliative care were introduced into the curricula of medical and nursing schools, and programmes about pain treatment were developed to provide continuous training for personnel in health-care facilities. At the same time, a number of regulatory reforms made it less difficult for opioids to be procured, prescribed and dispensed. Examples of such reform measures that have had a significant impact on the effective treatment of pain include extending the validity of prescriptions for opioid analgesics from 7 to 28 days and allowing nurses to administer opioids in the absence of a doctor. While promoting the consumption of opioids for the treatment of pain, the Government of France has, at the same time, established mechanisms to monitor and prevent the abuse and diversion of those substances. All of the above activities remained within the frame of the international conventions.

101. While increases in consumption levels for opioid analgesics may be easier to achieve in countries that, like France, have adequate resources for health care, such improvements are also possible in countries with more limited resources, such as Uganda. Over the past 10 years, morphine consumption in Uganda has increased steadily, as a result of the expansion of a programme that provides home-based palliative care to patients throughout the country. In Uganda, as in France, key factors in the successful implementation of this approach include the commitment of the Government to making relief from pain a health-care priority and the education of health-care professionals about the use of opioids and palliative care. Another important step towards ensuring access to morphine for patients in a range of health-care settings has been the introduction of legal reforms allowing nurses to prescribe morphine. That is an example of the kind of task-shifting recommended by WHO[26] to increase access to health-care services in situations where there is a shortage of health-care workers. Developing systems for the reliable procurement of morphine and

---

[26] World Health Organization, Task Shifting: Rational Redistribution of Tasks among Health Workforce Teams — Global Recommendations and Guidelines (Geneva, 2008).

making it available for oral administration, at a low cost, have also been essential to efforts to broaden access to that drug. Again all of the activities remained within the frame of the international conventions.

102. The examples of France and Uganda show that increased consumption of opioid analgesics can be achieved with strong governmental support through a multipronged strategy to remove impediments to their availability. Although many countries in Europe have consumption levels for opioids under international control that are comparable to that of France, a number of countries, including many in Eastern Europe, currently have levels of opioid consumption that are much lower than the level reported by France 10 years ago. For the majority of the people in many countries in Africa, access to low-cost oral morphine is practically non-existent. Unfortunately, inadequate access to opioids remains a reality in a large number of countries not only in Africa and Eastern Europe but in all regions. The Board calls upon the Governments of those countries to take determined steps to ensure adequate access to opioid analgesics and to reinforce the regulatory agencies, which is a key to adequate access to controlled drugs and their appropriate use. To that end, Governments should consider the recommendations contained in the 1995 special report of the Board on the availability of opiates for medical needs,[27] and in chapter I of the Board's report for 1999.

103. The Board notes with appreciation that in the past few years, the Governments of a number of countries, including Georgia, Guatemala, Panama, Serbia and Viet Nam, have introduced policy reforms aimed at ensuring adequate access to opioid analgesics. The Governments of those countries and others that are in the initial stages of developing strategies for improving the availability of opioids should provide strong support for the implementation of those strategies. Mechanisms should be in place for monitoring the implementation and the long-term effectiveness of policies to improve access to opioids.

104. The Board is of the opinion that there is an urgent need for some Governments to take specific measures to ensure that their populations have adequate access to opioid-based medications in accordance with the international drug control conventions. In particular, Governments of countries in which opioid consumption is below 100 S-DDD per million inhabitants per day and Governments of countries with no opioid consumption at all should immediately take appropriate action to ensure access to such medications. The key element is an effective regulatory body. It is not admissible that large parts of the world remain seriously undersupplied with medicines that are necessary to alleviate the pain and suffering of patients.

105. The Board calls the attention of Governments to the fact that accurate estimation of requirements for internationally controlled substances is essential to ensure the adequate availability of those substances for medical and scientific purposes. Poor estimation of those requirements can lead to many problems in the use of controlled substances in the health-care system, such as shortages, irrational prescribing, distortion of demand and low cost-effectiveness; it can also lead to surpluses and increased risk of diversion of controlled substances. Proper use of the system of estimates for narcotic drugs and the system of assessments for psychotropic substances is important to ensure adequate availability of internationally controlled substances. For this purpose, national

---

[27] Availability of Opiates for Medical Needs (see footnote 8 above).

competent authorities need to ensure that health-service providers can easily communicate their requirements to them.

B. Availability of internationally controlled substances above levels required for sound medical practice

106. Lack of availability of narcotic drugs and psychotropic substances may deprive patients of their fundamental rights and the opportunity to have relief from physical pain and from suffering due to mental illness. On the other hand, excessive availability of these drugs can lead to diversion and abuse and subsequently to drug dependence. Over recent years the Board has noted with increasing concern that the abuse of internationally controlled substances, diverted into illicit channels at various stages of their distribution, continues to be widespread in many countries and has in some countries reached or overtaken the levels of abuse of illicit drugs.

107. In a number of countries, the abuse of pharmaceuticals containing controlled substances is second only to the abuse of cannabis. The pharmaceutical preparations diverted and abused contain various opioids, benzodiazepines and amphetamine-type stimulants. Among opioids, diversion of preparations containing buprenorphine, codeine, dextropropoxyphene, fentanyl, hydrocodone, methadone, morphine, oxycodone and trimeperidine account for the largest quantities diverted. Among the psychotropic substances, alprazolam, buprenorphine, diazepam, flunitrazepam, phenobarbital and phentermine are the most often diverted and abused substances.

108. Data collected by Governments suggest that abuse patterns are related to excessive overall availability of the pharmaceutical preparations containing these substances. In particular, countries with already elevated levels of consumption of narcotic drugs and psychotropic substances that experience further significant increases should be vigilant to determine whether these increases are related to actual medical requirements or to their misuse and abuse. Changing drug prescription and drug consumption patterns is usually a slow process, and new drug consumption habits develop over a period of years. New fashions in drug abuse, on the other hand, develop quite fast, in particular when the drugs of abuse show the same effect as previously abused illicit drugs but are easier to obtain. A culture of widespread and excessive availability of pharmaceuticals that have effects similar to those created by illicit drugs will result in the increasing substitution of these pharmaceuticals for illicit drugs. Reversing such a trend is difficult and requires efforts, as the abused pharmaceuticals will remain available. This explains why, in countries with excessive availability, the non-medical use of pain relievers, tranquillizers, stimulants or sedatives has become the fastest-growing drug problem.

109. In most countries the problem of abuse of prescription drugs has received less attention from drug control regulators than abuse of illicit drugs. The systematic collection of data on prescription drug abuse in household surveys is at present carried out only in the United States, which means that reliable data on the extent of such abuse are limited to that country. The problem is, however, not restricted to the United States. Abuse of prescription drugs is reported from all regions in the world.

110. Abuse of prescription drugs can be as dangerous as abuse of illicit drugs. In particular, the share of prescription opioids in cases of death related to overdose has significantly increased. This has, unfortunately, been overlooked by the general public for a long time. Over the last decade the number of cases of death related to prescription drug abuse has risen significantly, overtaking in some countries the number of cases of death from overdose related to illicit drugs. However, it was only because the deaths of several prominent entertainers were related to abuse of prescription drugs that the media and the broader public have taken note of the dangers of prescription drug abuse. Action should be taken, however, before such high levels of abuse of prescription drugs are reached. Since excessive availability is often the first step towards increasing abuse of prescription drugs, drug control regulators need to be vigilant with regard to high consumption levels of narcotic drugs and psychotropic substances.

111. Increasing abuse of prescription drugs has led to rising levels of poly-drug addiction, combining licitly manufactured medicines and illicit drugs or several medicines containing internationally controlled substances. Equally, the abuse of combination products manufactured by the pharmaceutical industry or prescription formulas prepared in pharmacies combining several internationally controlled substances is increasing.

112. The Board encourages all Governments to identify unusual trends in consumption levels for narcotic drugs and psychotropic substances and to take remedial action, if required. In the absence of accepted norms for adequate consumption, Governments may wish to analyse past trends and compare their national consumption levels with those of other countries at a similar level of socio-economic development.

113. Such comparisons could be carried out on the basis of the tables on the consumption of opioid analgesics and the various groups of psychotropic substances published by the Board in its technical report on narcotic drugs and its technical report on psychotropic substances. The Governments of countries with particularly high or rising levels of consumption of narcotic drugs and psychotropic substances should monitor the situation closely, determine whether their territories are being used for illegally operating Internet pharmacies, identify possible overprescribing or any other unprofessional practices among medical professionals and ensure that domestic distribution channels are adequately controlled. All Governments should implement the recommendations of WHO on the rational prescribing of drugs and take measures to promote sound medical practices.[28]

114. To prevent substances under international control from being diverted in one country and subsequently smuggled into another, Governments should harmonize at the regional and subregional levels measures taken to reduce excessive consumption levels, so that the efforts made in one country will not result in problematic consumption patterns shifting to neighbouring countries.

115. However, the use of certain groups of substances may not differ only between countries with comparable levels of socio-economic development in different regions, but also between countries in

---

[28] "Promoting rational use of medicines: core components", *WHO Policy Perspectives on Medicines*, No. 5, September 2002. Available at http://whqlibdoc.who.int/hq/2002/WHO_EDM_2002.3.pdf.

the same region, owing to cultural and demographic factors. For example, significant cross-national and country-specific variations indicate considerable variances in medical practice between otherwise similar countries, and sometimes even within countries.

116. A persistent difference in consumption of internationally controlled substances is seen in the regional preferences for groups of psychotropic substances in Europe and in North America, two regions with similar levels of socio-economic development. While Europe records the world's top use of benzodiazepines, North America records the top consumption of performance-enhancing stimulants. This may imply cultural differences, but may also be related to demographics, as benzodiazepines are taken mostly by the older segments of the population, while performance- and body shape-enhancing drugs are consumed to a larger extent by adolescents and younger adults.

117. The channels of supply of abused prescription drugs vary, but, in principle, once they have left the officially controlled supply channels they are to be found in a "parallel market" of sometimes significant dimensions. In many countries, unregulated drug markets called "street markets" operate in parallel to or often in the absence of licensed pharmacies. The reasons for purchasing medications on such street markets are often related to economic factors or to an insufficient supply through official channels. Illegally operating Internet pharmacies are another kind of parallel market. As in street markets, customers can obtain internationally controlled drugs such as benzodiazepines, opioids, stimulants and barbiturates without a prescription. The supplies for these markets are often diverted or stolen products, or unregistered, substandard or counterfeit medications.

118. Depending on the country, the reasons for utilizing unregulated markets vary. They include limited access to health-care facilities, lower cost of drugs, which is often related to the fact that they are substandard or counterfeit products, overly stringent prescription requirements, the desire to obtain drugs without medical records to preserve privacy or demand for prescription drugs for abuse purposes.

119. All Governments should apply the International Narcotics Control Board guidelines for the control of Internet pharmacies,[29] because in some countries such pharmacies represent the principal channel for the illicit distribution of internationally controlled substances.

C. Ensuring adequate availability in emergency situations

120. Emergency situations in the wake of natural or man-made disasters may lead to a sudden and acute need for medicines containing controlled substances. Such a situation arose following the devastating earthquake in Haiti in January 2010. Controlled substances such as morphine and pentazocine were urgently required to provide medical care for the large number of people who had been injured in the earthquake.

---

[29] Guidelines for Governments on Preventing the Illegal Sale of Internationally Controlled Substances through the Internet (United Nations publication, Sales No. E.09.XI.6).

121. Humanitarian relief agencies have often found it difficult to rapidly obtain medicines containing controlled substances for medical care in emergency situations, in part because of the control measures exerted over the international movement of such medicines. The administrative requirements that must be fulfilled under normal circumstances to authorize the import and export of controlled substances slow down the supply of urgently needed medicines to disaster areas. This problem is compounded if competent national authorities in the importing countries are no longer functioning.

122. To address that issue, WHO, in consultation with the Board, prepared the Model Guidelines for the International Provision of Controlled Medicines for Emergency Medical Care.[30] The Guidelines provide a simplified procedure for the export of medicines containing controlled substances to be handled by reputable humanitarian relief agencies. Soon after the earthquake in Haiti, the Board sent letters to all Governments and selected humanitarian relief agencies to remind them about the simplified procedures contained in the Guidelines.

123. Because emergency situations come about suddenly, competent authorities should be prepared to use the simplified procedures contained in the Guidelines to expedite the supply of controlled medicines as soon as the need arises. The Board invites Governments and humanitarian relief agencies to bring to its attention any problems encountered in making deliveries of controlled medicines in emergency situations. Governments may wish to include in their special stocks of narcotic drugs and psychotropic substances quantities to meet the need for such substances in the event of an emergency situation.

---

[30] World Health Organization, document WHO/PSA/96.17.

VI. Conclusions and recommendations

124. The International Narcotics Control Board has frequently confirmed that the underlying principles of the international drug control treaties provide the mechanism to ensure availability of narcotic drugs and psychotropic substances for medical and scientific requirements while at the same time preventing their inappropriate use and abuse. Ensuring availability of narcotic drugs and psychotropic substances and preventing their diversion are not contradictory goals; in fact, action to achieve these two objectives can be in synergy if measures are correctly and fully implemented. The proper interpretation of these two complementary aims is accepted by an ever-wider range of countries. However, substantial progress is still required in a number of countries.

125. The Board notes that, in response to previous recommendations on availability of narcotic drugs, a significant number of Governments have increased their estimates to meet medical demand, issued national policies to improve medical use of narcotic drugs, supported educational programmes and examined their health-care systems, laws and regulations for impediments. There have been improvements in the adequacy of supply of certain narcotic drugs and psychotropic substances in many countries, but there have been setbacks in others. While the most significant improvements are recorded in highly developed countries, the setbacks, unfortunately, have occurred mostly in the regions that 20 years ago had the lowest levels of availability of internationally controlled substances.

126. As shown in the Board's analysis, a large number of countries in many regions continue to record inadequate levels of availability of internationally controlled substances. Africa remains the region with the largest number of countries recording little or no availability. Other regions where the situation has not improved, and in certain cases worsened, are Central America and the Caribbean and South Asia. However, even in regions with overall increasing levels of availability, countries remaining at the lower margin in terms of consumption of controlled substances record inadequately low levels of availability.

127. Among the countries with particularly low levels of availability are a number of countries with large populations; thus, large parts of the world population have no access to narcotic drugs and psychotropic substances. Also, even if countries have recorded improvements, the improvements may not have led to levels that could be considered adequate, because of low starting levels. In spite of the progress made towards meeting treaty objectives, relatively few countries in the world have an adequate drug supply management system and working mechanisms that ensure reliable, needs-based assessments, equitable availability and cost-effectiveness.

128. According to the analysis of the Board, deficiencies in drug supply management remain attributable to lack of financial resources, inadequate infrastructure, the low priority given to health

care, weak government authority, inadequate education and professional training, and outdated knowledge, which together affect the availability of not only controlled drugs but all medicines.

129. Substantial improvement in the availability of narcotic drugs and psychotropic substances is linked to progress in the availability of medicines in general, particularly in countries with limited resources for health, where growing economic disparities, pressing basic needs and poor infrastructure are the principal barriers to any lasting improvement. During recent years international awareness has increased, and efforts to facilitate the supply of licit drugs to underdeveloped areas are carried out by intergovernmental and non-governmental organizations. However, despite growing global awareness of the prevailing unsatisfactory situation, a considerable number of countries continue to show no appreciation of the problem itself or of the relative ease with which efficient treatment can be provided.

130. It appears that a number of countries have not yet recognized that adequate availability of medicines, including narcotic drugs and psychotropic substances, is an essential part of their responsibility towards their populations. Negligence towards this responsibility is shown when countries do not even estimate their requirements and appear to have no knowledge about the quantities of certain drugs their populations would require for medical treatment. In other countries, where such negligence is not observed, other obstacles continue to prevail, including outdated restrictive regulations and, more frequently, uninformed interpretations of otherwise correct regulations, misguided fears and ingrained prejudices about using opioids for medical purposes.

131. The Board has always emphasized that the efforts to limit the use of narcotic drugs and psychotropic substances to medical and scientific purposes must not adversely affect their availability for such purposes. On the other hand, increasing the use of certain controlled drugs for legitimate medical purposes needs thorough monitoring. Careful attention has to be given to ensuring the legitimate absorption capacity of countries and the proper functioning of safeguard mechanisms in order to minimize misuse and leaks in the system. The Board is of the opinion that a well-educated and functioning control-system administration is a prerequisite for ensuring availability, as it will be able to determine the quantities required and will identify shortages and problems in distribution. A functioning control-system administration will also be a responsible partner for cooperation with professional and consumer associations.

132. The overall goal of a well-functioning national and international system for managing the availability of narcotic drugs and psychotropic substances should be to provide relief from pain and suffering by ensuring the safe delivery of the best affordable drugs to those patients who need them and, at the same time, to prevent the diversion of drugs for the purpose of abuse. To ensure this, Governments need to fulfil the following essential tasks:

Recommendations on availability of narcotic drugs and psychotropic substances

(a) Governments should assess the actual requirements of the national health systems for internationally controlled substances; calculate their annual requirements for such substances and furnish the Board with timely estimates for narcotic drugs and assessments for psychotropic substances. In case national requirements are at the lower margin of levels of requirements in the region, Governments may need to critically examine their methods for assessing their medical requirements for narcotic drugs and psychotropic substances;

(b) Governments should identify impediments to availability of narcotic drugs and psychotropic substances (policy, regulatory, administrative) and take detailed, step-by-step measures to remove those impediments;

(c) Governments should establish a system to collect information from medical facilities that provide care for the mentally ill, addicts and surgery, cancer and other patients, from organizations that are working to improve the appropriate use of narcotic drugs and psychotropic substances, and should establish groups of knowledgeable individuals to assist in obtaining information about changing medical needs; they should also make use of available guidelines on assessing the actual requirements for narcotic drugs and psychotropic substances for their country;

(d) Once a country has reached an appropriate level of consumption of narcotic drugs and psychotropic substances, Governments should add to their annual estimates of requirements for narcotic drugs and assessments for psychotropic substances a margin to allow for the possibility of increased consumption from such general causes as population growth, evolution of health services and trends in the incidence of diseases and their treatment and, if need be, should add an even greater margin in countries or territories where there is rapid economic and social development or rapid expansion of the medical use of drugs, including the introduction of new formulations or drugs;

(e) Governments that experience interruptions in the supply of narcotic drugs and psychotropic substances because of delays in importation or for other reasons should examine the situation and develop a system to accomplish in a timely manner the steps involved, such as issuing licences, arranging for payment, carrying out paperwork, transporting the drugs, taking the drugs through customs and distributing the drugs to medical facilities;

(f) Governments should determine whether their national narcotics laws contain elements of the 1961 Convention as amended by the 1972 Protocol that take into account the fact that the medical use of narcotic drugs continues to be indispensable for the relief of pain and suffering and the fact that adequate provision must be made to ensure the availability of narcotic drugs for such purposes and to ensure that administrative responsibility has been established and that personnel are available for the implementation of those laws;

(g) Governments should determine whether there are undue restrictions in national narcotics laws, regulations or administrative policies that impede the prescribing or dispensing of, or needed medical treatment of patients with, narcotic drugs or psychotropic substances, or their availability and distribution for such purposes, and, should this be the case, make the necessary adjustments;

(h) To promote adequate availability of psychotropic substances globally and in specific countries pursuant to Commission on Narcotic Drugs resolution 53/4, Governments should collect the most reliable statistical data on the consumption of psychotropic substances and submit that information to the Board in timely fashion;

(i) Governments should fully cooperate with the Board in ensuring adequate availability of narcotic drugs and psychotropic substances; they should examine their medical needs for narcotic drugs and psychotropic substances, as well as the impediments to their availability, advise the Board of the results of those efforts and inform the Board if it can be of assistance; they should also inform the Board about progress and needs concerning implementation of the present recommendations;

Recommendations on appropriate use

(j) Governments should ensure the correct education and training of health professionals and should inform health professionals about the WHO analgesic method for cancer pain relief; they should communicate with health professionals about the legal requirements for prescribing and dispensing narcotic drugs and psychotropic substances and should provide an opportunity to discuss mutual concerns;

(k) Governments should ensure that comprehensive curricula on substance abuse and rational use of psychoactive drugs are used in relevant faculties of universities, medical, pharmaceutical and nursing schools and other health-care institutes;

(l) Governments should stimulate, through regulation and monitoring, ethical behaviour in drug marketing; they should ensure high professional standards in therapy (diagnosis, deciding on therapy, prescribing);

(m) Governments should educate the public in the appropriate use of narcotic drugs and psychotropic substances and in the correct use of pharmacotherapy with other therapeutic options, and should enlist in this effort the active participation of professional organizations and consumer associations;

(n) Governments should establish a comprehensive registration and authorization system and select carefully and support safer and more cost-effective drugs and reliable alternative treatment modalities;

(o) Governments should also encourage the development and use of better and safer therapeutic agents (with little or no dependence potential) to replace medicines with limited efficacy and safety. Countries experiencing abuse problems with regard to combination products or prescription formulas have a responsibility to make sure that action is taken to prevent such abuse;

Recommendations on national control systems

(p) Governments should endeavour to keep the supply and consumption of internationally controlled substances under close supervision. Experience has shown that particular attention needs to be given to adequate legislation and correct administrative arrangements, adapted, as required, to new trends and developments;

(q) Governments should establish a sufficient degree of government authority and regulatory control over the national drug supply, including the control of narcotic drugs and psychotropic substances;

(r) Governments should conduct inspections of manufacturers, exporters, importers and wholesale and retail distributors, as well as of stocks and records, and take appropriate action against those who fail to comply with applicable legal requirements and professional codes of conduct. Activities of market intermediaries such as brokers must be regulated, as appropriate;

(s) Governments need to ensure adequate financial and human resources for their drug regulatory authorities and other agencies and provide capacity-building to their staff;

(t) Governments need to implement effective policies to combat counterfeit drugs and provide a comprehensive legal framework to make trading in counterfeit products a serious criminal offence; exporting countries must regulate the process with a view to preventing the export of drugs that are counterfeit or of poor quality;

(u) Governments should be aware and make the best use of the Model Guidelines for the International Provision of Controlled Medicines for Emergency Medical Care;

Recommendations on prevention of diversion and abuse

(v) Governments should enforce existing legislation to ensure that narcotic drugs and psychotropic substances are not illegally manufactured, imported or exported and are not diverted to the unregulated market;

(w) Governments should collect data on the abuse of prescription drugs in a more systematic manner and include in their national surveys on drug abuse, as far as possible, pharmaceuticals containing narcotic drugs and psychotropic substances, by including either specific groups of substances or specific narcotic drugs and psychotropic substances, as required;

(x) Considering the international nature of the problem and to complement the efforts of law enforcement in individual countries in the above-mentioned areas, Governments, as well as regional and international organizations, should develop intergovernmental agreements for effective joint operations and arrangements and standards to be applied at the regional level;

(y) Governments should take prompt and effective action to implement previous recommendations of the Board on Internet trading and on the misuse of the mail for smuggling of internationally controlled substances.

133. To achieve the goal of adequate availability of narcotic drugs and psychotropic substances globally, support from the world community is required. Progress in countries with low levels of consumption of such drugs is usually gradual. Prevailing market conditions and the present supply system do not make it possible to ensure the availability of needed medicines in low-income

countries. Economic and financial conditions in such countries and insufficient health-care infrastructure are impediments that cannot be overcome by those countries alone. Progress can be achieved only on the basis of a more humanitarian approach that is in line with the treaty system. Such an approach in selected countries may include the provision of assistance in establishing more reliable baseline estimates and assessments of medical needs and consultations with potential suppliers under preferential conditions.

134. The Board concludes that if the above recommendations are implemented, there will be significant additional progress towards ensuring adequate availability of narcotic drugs and psychotropic substances for medical and scientific purposes. The Board will continue its examination of the situation and will monitor responses to its recommendations. To support progress the Board will continue to:

(a) Monitor annual estimates for narcotic drugs and assessments for psychotropic substances submitted by Governments and initiate dialogue as necessary to identify unmet needs and ensure that annual estimates or assessments of requirements for narcotic drugs and psychotropic substances are neither overestimated nor underestimated;

(b) Ensure expeditious confirmation of supplementary estimates and processing of modified assessments for psychotropic substances submitted by Governments to assist them in coping with unforeseeable needs;

(c) Review on a regular basis national and international developments relevant to improving the availability of narcotic drugs and psychotropic substances for medical purposes, incorporating updated information and observations into its annual report;

(d) Encourage Governments to develop drug distribution systems that are well controlled and that will ensure availability of narcotic drugs and psychotropic substances to patients in medical facilities and in the community;

(e) Cooperate with UNODC to include in the model national legislation on the control of narcotic drugs and psychotropic substances provisions that recognize the obligation to ensure the adequate availability of narcotic drugs and psychotropic substances for medical and scientific purposes;

(f) Respond to the call of the Commission on Narcotic Drugs in the area of availability of internationally controlled substances and support the Commission in its efforts to remind parties to the 1961 Convention and the 1971 Convention of their obligations in this respect;

(g) Cooperate with WHO to assist Governments in developing adequately controlled drug distribution systems that are capable of providing narcotic drugs and psychotropic substances to patients in hospitals and in the community;

(h) Alert the international community to new trends in abuse of pharmaceutical preparations containing narcotic drugs and psychotropic substances;

(i) Alert the international community to emerging new methods of trafficking of internationally controlled substances;

(j) Support Governments in implementing the provisions of the international drug control treaties and additional control measures, as requested by the Economic and Social Council, as well as the relevant guidelines of the Board.

Annex I

Tables on consumption of opioid analgesics in regions

Table 1
Levels of consumption of narcotic drugs: average consumption of narcotic drugs, 2007-2009, by region per day
(Defined daily doses for statistical purposes per million inhabitants per day)

Region	Codeine	Fentanyl	Hydro-codone	Hydro-morphone	Morphine	Oxycodone	Pethidine	Others	Total
Americas	31	3 781	6 850	337	809	2 217	40	254	**14 320**
North America	*58*	*7 481*	*13 738*	*675*	*1 564*	*4 441*	*72*	*509*	***28 536***
South America	*5*	*120*	*8*	*1*	*68*	*8*	*10*	*2*	***221***
Central America and the Caribbean	*<<*	*32*	*4*	*<<*	*16*	*4*	*8*	*1*	***65***
Oceania	70	2 727	<<	42	1 050	1 590	28	3	**5 510**
Europe	32	3 707	6	104	398	288	11	689	**5 236**
Asia	2	72	1	<<	14	7	5	4	**105**
West Asia	*2*	*123*	*-*	*<<*	*8*	*8*	*7*	*7*	***155***
East and South-East Asia	*3*	*102*	*<<*	*1*	*19*	*4*	*11*	*8*	***146***
South Asia	*<<*	*3*	*1*	*-*	*7*	*<<*	*1*	*4*	***17***
Africa	4	22	<<	<<	10	<<	3	11	**50**

Note: The symbol "<<" indicates an amount less than 1 defined daily dose for statistical purposes per million inhabitants per day.

Table 2
Levels of consumption of narcotic drugs

A. Average consumption of narcotic drugs in North America, South America and Central America and the Caribbean, 2007-2009
(Defined daily doses for statistical purposes per million inhabitants per day)

Regional ranking	Ranking in the Americas	World ranking	Country or non-metropolitan territory	Codeine	Fentanyl	Hydro-codone	Hydro-morphone	Morphine	Oxycodone	Pethidine	Others	Total
North America												
1	1	1	United States of America	<<	9 904	20 066	673	2 060	5 962	88	734	**39 487**
2	2	2	Canada	783	9 432	253	2 909	2 080	4 932	151	92	**20 632**
3	21	91	Mexico[a]	-	74	-	1	9	1	-	-	**85**
			Regional average: North America	58	7 481	13 738	675	1 564	4 441	72	509	**28 536**
South America												
1	3	20	Falkland Islands (Malvinas)[a]	369	2 347	-	-	452	-	31	1 084	**4 283**
2	6	52	Argentina	14	103	42	-	250	12	2	20	**443**
3	8	55	Chile	69	198	-	-	108	5	7	1	**388**
4	9	57	Colombia	-	188	34	4	42	24	1	-	**295**
5	12	61	Brazil	<<	139	-	-	59	3	17	-	**218**
6	13	71	Uruguay	-	77	1	-	76	-	10	-	**164**
7	23	97	Venezuela (Bolivarian Republic of)	-	47	-	<<	9	14	1	-	**71**
8	25	105	Ecuador	-	50	-	-	7	5	-	-	**62**
9	26	106	Suriname	27	12	-	-	18	-	4	-	**61**
10	27	107	Peru	-	26	-	-	19	9	4	-	**58**
11	31	119	Paraguay	-	28	-	-	2	-	8	-	**38**
12	33	146	Guyana	2	4	-	-	3	-	1	-	**10**
13	34	159	Bolivia (Plurinational State of)	-	<<	-	-	1	2	-	-	**3**
			Regional average: South America	5	120	8	1	68	8	10	2	**221**
Central America and the Caribbean												
1	4	29	Cayman Islands	18	1 465	181	32	89	714	408	2	**2 909**
2	5	41	Netherlands Antilles	-	1 080	-	-	82	2	20	45	**1 229**
3	7	54	Turks and Caicos Islands	2	133	-	-	10	151	57	39	**392**
4	10	58	Bahamas	8	8	-	-	40	96	140	-	**292**
5	11	59	Montserrat	223	<<	-	-	14	-	35	-	**272**
6	14	76	Trinidad and Tobago[a]	-	17	-	-	42	-	78	-	**137**
7	15	79	Panama	-	104	-	-	7	-	8	-	**119**
8	16	83	Costa Rica	-	41	-	-	61	-	2	-	**104**
9	17	84	Saint Lucia	29	1	4	-	21	-	36	-	**91**
10	18	85	El Salvador	-	48	3	-	4	19	16	-	**90**
11	19	87	Cuba	-	44	-	-	36	-	6	2	**88**

ANNEX I

Regional ranking	Ranking in the Americas	World ranking	Country or non-metropolitan territory	Codeine	Fentanyl	Hydro-codone	Hydro-morphone	Morphine	Oxycodone	Pethidine	Others	Total
12	20	89	Jamaica	2	14	-	-	30	-	40	-	86
13	21	91	Saint Vincent and the Grenadines	1	5	-	-	30	-	49	-	85
14	24	103	Grenada	7	4	-	-	14	-	31	7	63
15	28	114	Guatemala	-	16	21	-	4	4	3	<<	48
16	29	115	Dominica	-	1	-	-	7	-	38	-	46
17	30	118	Nicaragua	-	30	-	-	7	2	<<	-	39
18	32	129	Dominican Republic	-	15	-	-	8	1	<<	-	24
19	35	165	Haiti	<<	1	-	-	1	-	<<	-	2
Regional average: Central America and the Caribbean				<<	32	4	<<	16	4	8	1	65
Average: Americas				31	3 781	6 850	337	809	2 217	40	254	14 320

Notes: The symbol "<<" indicates an amount less than 1 defined daily dose for statistical purposes per million inhabitants per day.

As at 1 November 2010, in North America, the following territory had not submitted any statistical forms for the three consecutive years in question: *Bermuda*; in Central America and the Caribbean, the following eight countries and territories did either not submit any statistical forms or did not provide any consumption data for the three consecutive years in question: *Anguilla*, Antigua and Barbuda, *Aruba*, Barbados, Belize, *British Virgin Islands*, Honduras and Saint Kitts and Nevis.

[a] Calculation is based on data covering two years only.

B. Average consumption of narcotic drugs in Oceania, 2007-2009

(Defined daily doses for statistical purposes per million inhabitants per day)

Regional ranking	World ranking	Country or non-metropolitan territory	Codeine	Fentanyl	Hydrocodone	Hydromorphone	Morphine	Oxycodone	Pethidine	Others	Total
1	13	Australia	108	4 058	<<	64	1 381	2 367	31	4	8 013
2	24	Norfolk Island	42	2 740	-	-	393	213	15	-	3 403
3	32	New Caledonia	-	2 187	-	17	266	9	-	-	2 479
4	33	New Zealand	-	637	-	<<	1 192	479	56	<<	2 364
5	36	Wallis and Futuna Islands	135	823	-	-	18	-	-	1 161	2 137
6	38	French Polynesia	-	1 263	-	7	141	6	1	-	1 418
7	40	Christmas Island	9	818	-	-	12	487	8	-	1 334
8	51	Palau	34	2	485	-	16	-	27	-	564
9	81	Cook Islands[a]	-	-	-	-	41	-	66	-	107
10	88	Tonga[a]	50	3	-	-	15	-	19	-	87
11	111	Nauru[b]	5	13	-	-	14	-	21	-	53
12	120	Marshall Islands[b]	-	7	-	-	15	-	11	-	33
13	123	Papua New Guinea[b]	1	<<	-	-	15	-	15	-	31
		Vanuatu[b]	8	12	-	-	11	-	-	-	31
15	136	Samoa	-	1	-	-	7	-	7	-	15
Regional average: Oceania			70	2 727	<<	42	1 050	1 590	28	3	5 510

Notes: The symbol "<<" indicates an amount less than 1 defined daily dose for statistical purposes per million inhabitants per day.
As at 1 November 2010, the following six countries and territories either had not submitted any statistical forms or had not provided any consumption data for the three consecutive years in question: *Cocos (Keeling) Islands*, Fiji, Kiribati, Micronesia (Federated States of), Solomon Islands and Tuvalu.
[a] Calculation is based on data covering two years only.
[b] Calculation is based on data covering one year only.

C. Average consumption of narcotic drugs in Europe, 2007-2009
(Defined daily doses for statistical purposes per million inhabitants per day)

Regional ranking	World ranking	Country or non-metropolitan territory	Codeine	Fentanyl	Hydrocodone	Hydromorphone	Morphine	Oxycodone	Pethidine	Others	Total
1	3	Germany	1	12 772	41	615	619	836	14	4 421	**19 319**
2	4	Austria	17	10 252	-	932	4 593	200	6	160	**16 160**
3	5	Belgium	22	10 613	42	126	366	72	13	3 460	**14 714**
4	6	Denmark	-	8 078	6	74	1 523	2 298	75	992	**13 046**
5	7	Switzerland	98	7 649	67	232	1 238	717	80	2 963	**13 044**
6	8	Iceland	4 818	5 607	-	48	919	249	8	841	**12 490**
7	9	*Gibraltar*	-	10 714	-	-	325	37	15	44	**11 135**
8	10	Netherlands	-	6 460	-	31	377	470	9	839	**8 186**
9	11	Spain	-	7 702	-	53	180	107	22	8	**8 072**
10	12	Finland	35	6 861	-	17	107	1 023	3	12	**8 058**
11	14	Norway	16	5 284	6	12	810	1 225	32	241	**7 626**
12	15	Luxembourg	3	5 266	<<	120	197	2	4	1 431	**7 023**
13	16	Sweden	-	4 763	<<	200	584	1 074	3	192	**6 816**
14	17	France	129	5 055	-	43	1 024	328	1	184	**6 764**
15	18	Slovenia	59	4 726	-	172	761	308	6	236	**6 268**
16	19	Ireland	-	4 413	2	111	269	525	24	<<	**5 344**
17	21	Greece	<<	4 217	-	<<	14	<<	18	21	**4 270**
18	22	United Kingdom	1	1 281	<<	36	1 114	914	33	276	**3 655**
19	25	Hungary	24	2 925	<<	57	36	19	5	300	**3 366**
20	26	Czech Republic	60	2 444	-	117	142	193	37	64	**3 057**
21	27	Slovakia	3	2 884	-	32	37	51	8	6	**3 021**
22	28	Italy	-	2 479	-	26	78	118	5	220	**2 926**
23	30	Croatia	397	2 121	-	9	51	30	4	<<	**2 612**
24	31	Poland	221	2 055	-	<<	171	1	20	23	**2 491**
25	34	Andorra	-	2 203	-	-	74	71	13	-	**2 361**
26	35	Portugal	89	1 454	-	6	601	-	11	5	**2 166**
27	37	Serbia	<<	1 285	-	21	21	<<	2	494	**1 823**
28	42	Lithuania	<<	999	-	-	75	<<	19	<<	**1 093**
29	44	Montenegro	-	919	-	-	3	-	2	3	**927**
30	45	Latvia	2	734	-	-	57	7	6	14	**820**
31	46	Estonia	<<	555	-	-	112	113	24	1	**805**
32	47	Cyprus	-	474	-	-	72	81	39	-	**666**
33	48	Bosnia and Herzegovina	1	460	-	-	17	-	<<	140	**618**
34	53	Bulgaria	-	95	-	-	197	31	8	81	**412**
35	56	Malta	<<	67	-	<<	239	-	53	2	**361**
36	69	Romania	-	93	-	1	34	40	5	-	**173**
37	74	Belarus	-	118	-	-	14	-	-	24	**156**
38	81	Russian Federation	<<	75	-	-	12	-	-	20	**107**

REPORT ON THE AVAILABILITY OF INTERNATIONALLY CONTROLLED DRUGS

Regional ranking	World ranking	Country or non-metropolitan territory	Codeine	Fentanyl	Hydrocodone	Hydromorphone	Morphine	Oxycodone	Pethidine	Others	Total
39	98	Albania	-	28	-	-	20	-	3	18	69
40	101	Republic of Moldova	-	30	-	-	27	-	-	9	66
41	122	Ukraine	13	11	-	-	6	-	-	2	32
42	127	The former Yugoslav Republic of Macedonia	-	25	-	-	1	-	-	-	26
Regional average: Europe			32	3 707	6	104	398	288	11	689	**5 236**

Note: The symbol "<<" indicates an amount less than 1 defined daily dose for statistical purposes per million inhabitants per day.

D. Average consumption of narcotic drugs in East and South-East Asia, South Asia and West Asia, 2007-2009

(Defined daily doses for statistical purposes per million inhabitants per day)

Regional ranking	Ranking in Asia	World ranking	Country or non-metropolitan territory	Codeine	Fentanyl	Hydrocodone	Hydromorphone	Morphine	Oxycodone	Pethidine	Others	Total
East and South-East Asia												
1	2	39	Republic of Korea	15	1 079	16	26	50	128	15	13	1 342
2	3	43	Japan	25	805	-	-	76	98	3	16	1 023
3	6	62	*Hong Kong, China*	<<	89	2	<<	86	<<	20	11	208
4	7	63	Singapore	<<	127	<<	-	31	20	19	<<	197
5	13	73	*Macao, China*	-	100	-	-	42	<<	16	<<	158
6	15	80	Malaysia	-	60	-	-	33	5	18	<<	116
7	16	86	Brunei Darussalam	-	34	-	-	33	-	20	2	89
8	19	99	China	2	37	<<	<<	17	2	10	<<	68
9	20	100	Thailand	<<	36	-	-	23	-	8	-	67
10	23	110	Mongolia	2	6	-	-	47	-	-	1	56
11	26	125	Democratic People's Republic of Korea	7	-	-	-	23	-	-	-	30
12	27	126	Viet Nam	-	17	-	-	8	-	4	-	29
13	35	145	Philippines	-	4	-	<<	4	2	1	-	11
14	36	148	Indonesia	-	6	-	-	1	-	2	-	9
15	41	157	Cambodia	1	3	-	-	2	-	<<	-	6
16	43	159	Lao People's Democratic Republic[a]	-	1	<<	-	<<	-	2	-	3
17	47	179	Myanmar	<<	<<	-	-	<<	-	<<	<<	<<
	Regional average: East and South-East Asia			3	102	<<	1	19	4	11	8	146
South Asia												
1	28	127	Sri Lanka	-	3	-	-	16	-	7	-	26
2	29	130	Bhutan[b]	7	1	-	-	3	-	10	-	21
3	30	134	India	-	4	1	-	8	<<	<<	4	17
4	34	144	Maldives[a]	-	3	-	-	4	-	5	-	12
5	36	148	Nepal	-	1	-	-	6	-	2	-	9
6	40	153	Bangladesh[a]	-	1	-	-	1	-	5	-	7
	Regional average: South Asia			<<	3	1	-	7	<<	1	4	17
West Asia												
1	1	23	Israel	86	2 719	-	2	140	500	26	9	3 482
2	4	50	Turkey	-	513	-	-	23	-	15	44	595
3	5	60	Bahrain	2	131	-	-	47	-	51	-	231
4	8	64	Saudi Arabia[a]	22	132	-	1	16	2	22	<<	195

REPORT ON THE AVAILABILITY OF INTERNATIONALLY CONTROLLED DRUGS

Regional ranking	Ranking in Asia	World ranking	Country or non-metropolitan territory	Codeine	Fentanyl	Hydrocodone	Hydromorphone	Morphine	Oxycodone	Pethidine	Others	Total
5	9	65	Kuwait	6	126	-	<<	13	5	41	-	191
6	10	66	Jordan	-	111	-	<<	43	-	32	-	186
7	11	67	Lebanon	-	125	-	-	35	-	24	1	185
8	12	68	United Arab Emirates	<<	143	-	4	14	3	11	4	179
9	14	75	Qatar	1	100	-	-	27	1	22	2	153
10	17	94	Georgia	<<	33	-	-	39	-	-	2	74
11	18	96	Syrian Arab Republic	-	23	-	-	3	35	11	-	72
12	21	102	Kazakhstan	<<	40	-	-	4	-	-	20	64
13	22	103	Oman	1	33	-	-	19	-	10	<<	63
14	24	115	Iran (Islamic Republic of)	-	28	-	-	-	-	18	-	46
15	25	117	Armenia	-	14	-	-	26	-	-	2	42
16	31	136	Azerbaijan	-	11	-	-	2	-	-	2	15
			Turkmenistan	<<	3	-	-	6	-	-	6	15
18	33	140	Kyrgyzstan	<<	9	-	-	2	-	-	3	14
19	36	148	Yemen	-	7	-	<<	1	-	1	-	9
20	39	151	Uzbekistan	<<	3	-	-	3	-	-	2	8
21	41	157	Iraq[b]	-	1	-	-	1	-	4	-	6
22	43	159	Pakistan	-	2	-	-	1	-	<<	-	3
			Tajikistan	<<	2	-	-	<<	-	-	1	3
24	46	174	Afghanistan[b]	-	<<	-	-	1	-	<<	-	1
Regional average: West Asia				2	123	-	<<	8	8	7	7	155
Average: Asia				2	72	1	<<	14	7	5	4	105

Notes: The symbol "<<" indicates an amount less than 1 defined daily dose for statistical purposes per million inhabitants per day.
As at 1 November 2010, in East and South-East Asia, the following country had not submitted any statistical forms for the three consecutive years in question: Timor-Leste.

[a] Calculation is based on data covering two years only.
[b] Calculation is based on data covering one year only.

E. Average consumption of narcotic drugs in Africa, 2007-2009
(Defined daily doses for statistical purposes per million inhabitants per day)

Regional ranking	World ranking	Country or non-metropolitan territory	Codeine	Fentanyl	Hydrocodone	Hydromorphone	Morphine	Oxycodone	Pethidine	Others	Total
1	49	South Africa	63	274	-	-	125	<<	32	106	600
2	70	*Saint Helena*	77	26	-	-	38	-	26	-	167
3	72	Algeria	-	26	-	-	3	-	<<	133	162
4	77	Tunisia	-	61	-	-	59	-	3	-	123
5	78	Seychelles	4	16	-	-	85	-	15	-	120
6	89	Libyan Arab Jamahiriya[a]	<<	62	-	-	1	-	23	-	86
7	93	Mauritius[a]	-	15	-	-	24	-	36	-	75
8	95	*Ascension Island*[a]	-	21	-	-	14	-	38	-	73
9	107	*Tristan da Cunha*[a]	-	-	-	-	55	-	3	-	58
10	109	Namibia	<<	22	-	-	27	-	7	1	57
11	112	Cape Verde	-	37	-	-	9	-	3	-	49
		Egypt	-	41	<<	<<	4	<<	4	-	49
13	120	Morocco	-	26	-	-	7	-	-	-	33
14	130	Botswana	-	1	-	-	15	-	5	<<	21
15	132	Uganda[a]	5	-	-	-	13	-	1	-	19
16	133	Zimbabwe[a]	-	1	-	-	6	-	8	3	18
17	135	Kenya	-	1	-	-	6	-	6	3	16
18	136	Ghana	-	<<	-	-	1	-	14	-	15
19	140	Zambia	-	<<	-	-	4	-	10	-	14
20	142	Madagascar	-	1	-	-	<<	-	-	12	13
		Malawi	<<	<<	-	-	5	-	8	-	13
22	146	Gabon[b]	-	10	-	-	<<	-	<<	-	10
23	151	Lesotho[a]	-	1	-	-	<<	-	7	-	8
24	153	Democratic Republic of the Congo	4	<<	-	-	2	-	<<	-	7
		Mozambique	-	2	-	-	4	-	1	-	7
		Sao Tome and Principe	-	7	-	-	<<	-	-	-	7
27	159	Mauritania[a]	-	3	-	-	<<	-	-	-	3
		Senegal[a]	-	1	-	-	2	-	-	-	3
29	165	Angola[a]	-	1	-	-	<<	-	<<	-	2
		Benin	-	1	-	-	<<	-	1	-	2
		Côte d'Ivoire	-	2	-	-	<<	-	-	-	2
		Eritrea	1	-	-	-	<<	-	1	-	2
		Ethiopia[a]	<<	<<	-	-	1	-	1	-	2
		Niger	<<	2	-	-	<<	-	<<	-	2
		Sierra Leone[b]	2	<<	-	-	<<	-	<<	-	2
		Togo	-	1	-	-	<<	-	1	-	2

REPORT ON THE AVAILABILITY OF INTERNATIONALLY CONTROLLED DRUGS

Regional ranking	World ranking	Country or non-metropolitan territory	Codeine	Fentanyl	Hydrocodone	Hydromorphone	Morphine	Oxycodone	Pethidine	Others	Total
37	174	Burkina Faso	-	1	-	-	<<	-	<<	-	1
		Burundi[a]	<<	<<	-	-	<<	-	1	-	1
		Comoros[b]	-	-	-	-	<<	-	1	-	1
		Sudan	-	<<	-	-	<<	-	1	-	1
41	179	Cameroon[a]	-	<<	-	-	<<	-	<<	<<	<<
		Chad[b]	-	<<	-	-	<<	-	<<	-	<<
		Mali[a]	-	<<	-	-	<<	-	-	-	<<
		Nigeria	-	<<	-	-	<<	-	<<	-	<<
		Rwanda	-	<<	-	-	<<	-	<<	-	<<
		United Republic of Tanzania	-	-	-	-	<<	-	-	<<	<<
Regional average: Africa			4	22	<<	<<	10	<<	3	11	50

Notes: The symbol "<<" indicates an amount less than 1 defined daily dose for statistical purposes per million inhabitants per day.

As at 1 November 2010, the following 10 countries either had not submitted any statistical forms or had not provided any consumption data for the three consecutive years in question: Central African Republic, Congo, Djibouti, Equatorial Guinea, Gambia, Guinea, Guinea-Bissau, Liberia, Somalia and Swaziland.

[a] Calculation is based on data covering two years only.
[b] Calculation is based on data covering one year only.

Annex II

Joint letter from the President of the International Narcotics Control Board and the Chair of the United Nations Development Group

UNITED NATIONS   **NATIONS UNIES**

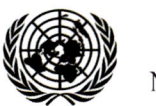

24 August 2001

Dear Colleagues,

As Resident Coordinator of the UN system at the country level, you are called upon, from time to time, to support the work and raise the concerns of UN bodies and organizations. We are writing to you to seek your support and assistance with regard to some of the issues and concerns important to the International Narcotics Control Board (INCB).

The INCB is the independent and quasi-judicial organ that monitors the implementation of the international drug control treaties. The Board is a treaty body established by the Single Convention on Narcotic Drugs of 1961, and its thirteen members are elected by ECOSOC to serve in their personal capacities, and not as representatives of their respective governments. The members of the Board come from different fields of expertise in dealing with the drug problem, and currently include senior police/law enforcement officials, former diplomats, veteran medical practitioners, noted researchers and the like. The 1961 Convention requires the UN Secretary-General to provide the Board with a secretariat, and the Secretary of the Board and his staff are therefore administratively part of the United Nations International Drug Control Programme (UNDCP) based in Vienna, Austria and report to the Board on all substantive issues. The Board's mandate under the Conventions is to limit to medical and scientific purposes the manufacture of, trade in and use of drugs. The Board is accordingly endowed with regulatory and quasi-judicial powers concerning the manufacture of, and trade in, medicaments containing internationally scheduled substances. The Board and its staff also monitor the international trade in chemicals frequently used in the illicit manufacture of drugs.

The Board's annual report for 1999 highlighted the under-consumption and the lack of medicaments available for the treatment of severe pain in many developing countries. Countries with a high incidence of cancer and AIDS, for example, are directly affected as essential medicines for the treatment of severe pain associated with such conditions are often not available. We therefore urge you to be aware of these issues when you establish your future priorities in programmes for the development of the health sector. We also urge you to raise this issue when you discuss health and development with government, the donor community and non-governmental organizations in your country of operation.

Further, the INCB undertakes periodic missions to our programme countries. The purpose of the missions, which generally comprise one or two Board members and a member of the Vienna-based secretariat, varies from country to country, and could range from encouraging accession to one or more of the international drug control treaties to close examination of the implementation of the treaties and fact finding. We urge each one of you to provide your full support to these missions, and to meet with the missions to discuss drug issues in your country of operation.

Finally, the Board launches an annual report, usually in late February, assessing the world drug situation in relation to the international drug control conventions and reporting on the activities of the preceding year. Your support for this event will be very much appreciated.

We look forward to your cooperation and participation, as the Resident Coordinator of the UN system at the country level, in these areas where our mutual expertise in development work and the international drug conventions can make a difference.

Mark Malloch Brown
Chair
United Nations Development Group

Hamid Ghodse
President
International Narcotics Control Board

Annex III

Follow-up joint letter from the President of the International Narcotics Control Board and the Chair of the United Nations Development Group

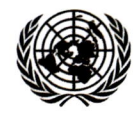

UNITED NATIONS   NATIONS UNIES

24 February 2005

Dear Resident Coordinators,

As Resident Coordinators of the UN system at the country level, you are called upon to support the work as well as raise the concerns of UN bodies and organizations. As was the case in 2001, we are again pleased to introduce the International Narcotics Control Board to you and to renew our call for your support and assistance with regard to the issues and concerns the Board addresses.

The INCB is a treaty body established by the Single Convention on Narcotic Drugs of 1961 that monitors the implementation of the international drug control treaties. It is an independent and quasi-judicial body composed of 13 members elected by ECOSOC to serve in their personal capacities, and not as representatives of their respective governments. The members of the Board are renowned experts of the different control fields. The present Board comprises senior law enforcement officials, former diplomats, veteran medical practitioners and pharmacists, demand reduction specialists, and noted academics and researchers.

The Board is assisted in its work by a secretariat provided by the UN Secretary-General, and headed by a Secretary. The Secretariat and the Secretary of the Board and his colleagues are administratively part of the United Nations Office on Drugs and Crime (UNODC) based in Vienna. However, the Secretary reports to the Board on all substantive issues.

The Board's mandate under the Convention is to limit to medical and scientific purposes the manufacture of, trade in and use of drugs. The Board is accordingly endowed with regulatory and quasi-judicial powers concerning the manufacture of, and trade in, medicaments containing internationally scheduled substances. Since the coming into force of the 1988 Convention, the Board also monitors the international trade in chemicals frequently used in the illicit manufacture of drugs.

The specific areas of cooperation we would request of you, as Resident Coordinators, include:

Field missions: To maintain dialogue at country level, the Board undertakes annually about 20 missions to different regions of the world. The purpose of the missions, which generally comprise one or two Board members accompanied by a staff of its Vienna-based secretariat, varies from country to country, but usually ranges from encouraging member States to accede to the international drug control treaties to close examination of the implementation of the treaties by governments.

The missions are generally prepared and organized from the logistical point of view in cooperation with governments and UNODC. However, in many places, your assistance is required either for arranging the mission or providing substantive briefing to INCB mission members on the drug situation in your country of operation.

Launch of INCB annual reports: The Board publishes an annual report on its work, which is launched usually in February. While this is done in cooperation with UNIS, you may be called upon to assist either at the request of the INCB or a government.

Dissemination of the findings of the Board: The findings in the Board reports are disseminated worldwide to the general public through national and international channels. You may be called upon by INCB to assist in this process.

Action-oriented programmes: The issues addressed by the Board serve as the basis for policy and action-oriented programmes in drug control and related matters. Examples of issues dealt with by the Board recently include the access and availability of drugs for medical use, especially in developing countries; illicit drugs and economic development and the complex relationship between drug abuse, crime and violence at the community level. As you can see, these issues are of direct relevance to UNDP's mandate. As Resident Representatives of UNDP and UN Resident Coordinators, we request you to consider their inclusion in your future priorities in development programmes, and to raise them when you discuss with government, the donor community and non-governmental organizations in your country of operation.

We look forward to your cooperation and participation, as the Resident Coordinator of the UN system at the country level, in these areas where our mutual expertise in development work and international drug control can make a difference.

Mark Malloch Brown
Chair
United Nations Development Group

Hamid Ghodse
President
International Narcotics Control Board

Annex IV

Letter from the President of the International Narcotics Control Board to all countries

UNITED NATIONS INTERNATIONAL NARCOTICS CONTROL BOARD

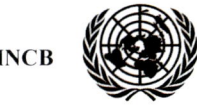

INCB OICS

NATIONS UNIES ORGANE INTERNATIONAL DE CONTRÔLE DES STUPÉFIANTS

Vienna International Centre, P.O. Box 500, A-1400 Vienna, Austria
Telephone: +43-1-26060, Telefax: +43-1-26060-5867/5868, Telex: 135612 uno a
E-Mail: secretariat@incb.org   Internet Address: http://www.incb.org/

Reference: INCB 114 (3) & 121 & 141
Decision: 84/53

24 April 2006
CU 2006/74

Excellency,

On behalf of the United Nations International Narcotics Control Board (INCB), I have the honour to refer to the responsibilities of the Board under the international drug control treaties, which are to promote Government compliance with those treaties and to monitor the functioning of the international control system.

With a history of nearly a century, the international drug control conventions are among the oldest international conventions ratified by most countries. National legislations are guided by these international obligations. The purpose of the conventions was to secure a balance between the appropriate use of narcotic drugs and psychotropic substances and their undesirable effects such as abuse and dependence. The cornerstone of the conventions is therefore to limit the use of these drugs and substances to medical and scientific purposes. Over recent years, the Board has brought to the attention of the governments that, in addition to international control of production/manufacture and international trade, there is a need for other aspects of prevention, particularly demand reduction, to be promoted and advanced, if substance abuse and dependence are going to be prevented.

Health care professionals can play an important role in these efforts by ensuring that the balance between benefit and risk is kept in mind and that the use of narcotic drugs and psychotropic substances is appropriate and in line with the pertinent recommendations of the World Health Organization (WHO) on the rational use of drugs. However, there are problems of access to these very effective drugs for needy patients due to a variety of reasons which were discussed in the Board's Report for 1999. Overuse of drugs in some countries creates other problems and this aspect was covered comprehensively in the Board's Report for 2000. For example, just six countries account for the use of 80% of licitly produced narcotic analgesics while 80% of the world's population have very little or no access to these drugs.

Universities are well placed to understand the different factors that affect health in relation to human development and to monitor ways in which such development can be used to enhance the quality of life. The Board therefore believes that the education and training of professionals involved in the caring professions and, as appropriate, of those in law and regulatory disciplines as well as social and behavioural sciences, is of the utmost importance. Universities clearly have a prominent role in leadership in this area, not only in research and advocacy, but also by ensuring that the relevant topics are included in undergraduate and postgraduate curricula.

The Board has requested me to bring these views to the attention of your Government. In particular, the Board wishes to encourage your Government to take measures to ensure the inclusion of the subject of the rational use of drugs for medical purposes and the risks associated with substance abuse and addictions to drugs in the curricula of the appropriate faculties in the universities, taking into account the need for coherent programmes in the various fields of study. Concerted action in this field could also cover misuse and abuse of alcohol and tobacco, although the Board has no mandate in these areas. The Board would respectfully request you to bring this to the attention of ministers of higher education, chancellors of the universities and other appropriate ministries, for their consideration.

The Board and its secretariat are happy to provide your Government and universities, with copies of INCB annual reports and publications to facilitate the development of such curricula.

I am attaching a brochure presenting the Board and its functions for your information.

Accept, Excellency, the assurance of my highest consideration.

Hamid Ghodse
President
International Narcotics Control Board

About the International Narcotics Control Board

The International Narcotics Control Board (INCB) is an independent and quasi-judicial control organ, established by treaty, for monitoring the implementation of the international drug control treaties. It had predecessors under the former drug control treaties as far back as the time of the League of Nations.

Composition

INCB consists of 13 members who are elected by the Economic and Social Council and who serve in their personal capacity, not as Government representatives. Three members with medical, pharmacological or pharmaceutical experience are elected from a list of persons nominated by the World Health Organization (WHO) and 10 members are elected from a list of persons nominated by Governments. Members of the Board are persons who, by their competence, impartiality and disinterestedness, command general confidence. The Council, in consultation with INCB, makes all arrangements necessary to ensure the full technical independence of the Board in carrying out its functions. INCB has a secretariat that assists it in the exercise of its treaty-related functions. The INCB secretariat is an administrative entity of the United Nations Office on Drugs and Crime, but it reports solely to the Board on matters of substance. INCB closely collaborates with the Office in the framework of arrangements approved by the Council in its resolution 1991/48. INCB also cooperates with other international bodies concerned with drug control, including not only the Council and its Commission on Narcotic Drugs, but also the relevant specialized agencies of the United Nations, particularly WHO. It also cooperates with bodies outside the United Nations system, especially the International Criminal Police Organization (INTERPOL) and the World Customs Organization.

Functions

The functions of INCB are laid down in the following treaties: the Single Convention on Narcotic Drugs of 1961 as amended by the 1972 Protocol; the Convention on Psychotropic Substances of 1971; and the United Nations Convention against Illicit Traffic in Narcotic Drugs and Psychotropic Substances of 1988. Broadly speaking, INCB deals with the following:

(a) As regards the licit manufacture of, trade in and use of drugs, INCB endeavours, in cooperation with Governments, to ensure that adequate supplies of drugs are available for medical and scientific uses and that the diversion of drugs from licit sources to illicit channels does not occur. INCB also monitors Governments' control over chemicals used in the illicit manufacture of drugs and assists them in preventing the diversion of those chemicals into the illicit traffic;

(b) As regards the illicit manufacture of, trafficking in and use of drugs, INCB identifies weaknesses in national and international control systems and contributes to correcting such situations. INCB is also responsible for assessing chemicals used in the illicit manufacture of drugs, in order to determine whether they should be placed under international control.

In the discharge of its responsibilities, INCB:

(a) Administers a system of estimates for narcotic drugs and a voluntary assessment system for psychotropic substances and monitors licit activities involving drugs through a statistical returns system, with a view to assisting Governments in achieving, inter alia, a balance between supply and demand;

(b) Monitors and promotes measures taken by Governments to prevent the diversion of substances frequently used in the illicit manufacture of narcotic drugs and psychotropic substances and assesses such substances to determine whether there is a need for changes in the scope of control of Tables I and II of the 1988 Convention;

(c) Analyses information provided by Governments, United Nations bodies, specialized agencies or other competent international organizations, with a view to ensuring that the provisions of the international drug control treaties are adequately carried out by Governments, and recommends remedial measures;

(d) Maintains a permanent dialogue with Governments to assist them in complying with their obligations under the international drug control treaties and, to that end, recommends, where appropriate, technical or financial assistance to be provided.

INCB is called upon to ask for explanations in the event of apparent violations of the treaties, to propose appropriate remedial measures to Governments that are not fully applying the provisions of the treaties or are encountering difficulties in applying them and, where necessary, to assist Governments in overcoming such difficulties. If, however, INCB notes that the measures necessary to remedy a serious situation have not been taken, it may call the matter to the attention of the parties concerned, the Commission on Narcotic Drugs and the Economic and Social

Council. As a last resort, the treaties empower INCB to recommend to parties that they stop importing drugs from a defaulting country, exporting drugs to it or both. In all cases, INCB acts in close cooperation with Governments.

INCB assists national administrations in meeting their obligations under the conventions. To that end, it proposes and participates in regional training seminars and programmes for drug control administrators.

Reports

The international drug control treaties require INCB to prepare an annual report on its work. The annual report contains an analysis of the drug control situation worldwide so that Governments are kept aware of existing and potential situations that may endanger the objectives of the international drug control treaties. INCB draws the attention of Governments to gaps and weaknesses in national control and in treaty compliance; it also makes suggestions and recommendations for improvements at both the national and international levels. The annual report is based on information provided by Governments to INCB, United Nations entities and other organizations. It also uses information provided through other international organizations, such as INTERPOL and the World Customs Organization, as well as regional organizations.

The annual report of INCB is supplemented by detailed technical reports. They contain data on the licit movement of narcotic drugs and psychotropic substances required for medical and scientific purposes, together with an analysis of those data by INCB. Those data are required for the proper functioning of the system of control over the licit movement of narcotic drugs and psychotropic substances, including preventing their diversion to illicit channels. Moreover, under the provisions of article 12 of the 1988 Convention, INCB reports annually to the Commission on Narcotic Drugs on the implementation of that article. That report, which gives an account of the results of the monitoring of precursors and of the chemicals frequently used in the illicit manufacture of narcotic drugs and psychotropic substances, is also published as a supplement to the annual report.

Since 1992, the first chapter of the annual report has been devoted to a specific drug control issue on which INCB presents its conclusions and recommendations in order to contribute to policy-related discussions and decisions in national, regional and international drug control. The following topics were covered in past annual reports:

1992: Legalization of the non-medical use of drugs
1993: The importance of demand reduction
1994: Evaluation of the effectiveness of the international drug control treaties
1995: Giving more priority to combating money-laundering
1996: Drug abuse and the criminal justice system
1997: Preventing drug abuse in an environment of illicit drug promotion
1998: International control of drugs: past, present and future
1999: Freedom from pain and suffering
2000: Overconsumption of internationally controlled drugs
2001: Globalization and new technologies: challenges to drug law enforcement in the twenty-first century
2002: Illicit drugs and economic development
2003: Drugs, crime and violence: the microlevel impact
2004: Integration of supply and demand reduction strategies: moving beyond a balanced approach
2005: Alternative development and legitimate livelihoods
2006: Internationally controlled drugs and the unregulated market
2007: The principle of proportionality and drug-related offences
2008: The international drug control conventions: history, achievements and challenges
2009: Primary prevention of drug abuse

Chapter I of the report of the International Narcotics Control Board for 2010 is entitled "Drugs and corruption".

Chapter II presents an analysis of the operation of the international drug control system based primarily on information that Governments are required to submit directly to INCB in accordance with the international drug control treaties. Its focus is on the worldwide control of all licit activities related to narcotic drugs and psychotropic substances, as well as chemicals used in the illicit manufacture of such drugs.

Chapter III presents some of the major developments in drug abuse and trafficking and measures by Governments to implement the international drug control treaties by addressing those problems.

Chapter IV presents the main recommendations addressed by INCB to Governments, the United Nations Office on Drugs and Crime, WHO and other relevant international and regional organizations.